Cover Image Credit/Copyright Attribution: IIerlok_Xolms/Shutterstock

Non-Communicable Disease Prevention

Best Buys, Wasted Buys and Contestable Buys

Edited by Wanrudee Isaranuwatchai, Rachel A. Archer, Yot Teerawattananon and Anthony J. Culyer

Contents

To those who are making a difference, and those who would like to make a difference in our healthcare system.

Forewords

The ultimate purpose of the Prince Mahidol Award Foundation under Royal Patronage, according to my interpretation, is to pursue the ideology of Prince Mahidol of Songkla in serving the benefit of mankind. The Foundation has three activities: the Prince Mahidol Award, the PMAC (Prince Mahidol Award Conference) and the Prince Mahidol Award Youth Program. The theme of PMAC 2019 was 'The Political Economy of NCDs: A Whole of Society Approach'. The idea to publish this book, *Non-communicable Disease Prevention: Best Buys, Wasted Buys and Contestable Buys*, was proposed during the PMAC 2019 preparation meeting and has been partially funded by PMAC.

PMAC is proud to have supported the development and dissemination of this book. In fact, it is more than just a book. We hope that it will be a collective learning tool for NCD managers and stakeholders, together with health economists or health intervention and technology assessment specialists. The ultimate goal of the learning process is 'good health at reasonable cost' with emphasis on NCDs. Taking a broader perspective, this learning process aims to help strengthen universal health coverage (UHC) schemes.

NCDs and their root causes are very complex; addressing or preventing them is even more complex. A policy or intervention which is thought to be Best Buy can turn out to be Wasted Buy. Even when there is evidence of high cost-effectiveness in one country, when the intervention is transferred directly to another country, it can become a Wasted Buy.

This is a book of evidence management and utilization in NCD prevention, which can be applied to the development of health systems as a whole. The key proposal is the SEED Tool (Systematic thinking for Evidence-based and Efficient Decision-making). To me, it is a framework or conceptualization tool that can handle complex situations. The decision-making process proposed is not linear, but a learning loop to guide deliberation. The book helps the target audience scrutinize evidence, mainly cost-effectiveness analyses, to be applied in local contexts with involvement.

PMAC is proud to present this high-quality commissioned work. We hope it will help to change the paradigm from communicable-disease-oriented health systems to more NCD-oriented systems, which is a much more complex paradigm.

Prof. Vicharn Panich
Chairperson of PMAC International Organizing Committee

Since 2007, the Prince Mahidol Award Conference (PMAC) has been organized as an annual international conference focusing on policy of global significance related to public health. For over a decade, PMAC has provided opportunities for debate, discussion and deliberation on priority global health policy and systems, and it has contributed to the exchange of knowledge and experience on global health between participants from across the world. In 2018, PMAC initiated commissioned work to provide a body of evidence to facilitate the sharing of experience at country level and among country and regional networks, in order to influence the implementation of global health and/or national policies and to enhance PMAC's capacities to deliver its knowledge and experiences to a wider spectrum of people.

Non-Communicable Disease Prevention: Best Buys, Wasted Buys and Contestable Buys is the first PMAC-commissioned work. This book provides evidence-informed insights to help understand which non-communicable disease (NCD) interventions work and which don't, so that program managers, policy officers and decision-makers in low- and middle-income countries (LMICs) can assess and implement interventions for the prevention and control of NCDs. It is a gold mine of very informative, easy to read and extremely helpful guidelines for those who wish to implement or reassess their strategies for preventing the NCD burden in their settings.

Non-Communicable Disease Prevention will augment PMAC's contribution in terms of changing health policy and improving health systems in different settings in relation to NCDs. It will continue the momentum of the PMAC 2019 theme on 'The Political Economy of NCDs: A Whole of Society Approach', enable the contributions from PMAC to reach a wider audience and sustain PMAC work into the future. This sharing of real world case studies, practical guidelines and key learning points will truly benefit all relevant stakeholders and the global health community and help accelerate the global progress in NCD prevention and control.

Prof. Churnrurtai Kanchanachitra
PMAC Secretariat

Demographic change, like climate change, proceeds slowly. National populations — starting from very different positions — exhibit a steady, usually predictable, but always slow increase in the number of individuals at older ages. The risks of stroke, heart disease, cancers and chronic respiratory illness increase sharply with age. Thus demography drives increases in incidence and mortality from these conditions. These changes — like the consequences of climate change — often remain below the threshold of visibility. Until they don't. Almost all middle-income countries (and many low-income ones) have crossed a threshold where the major non-communicable diseases (NCDs) have become highly salient in public discourse and, more practically, in the budgetary demands on health systems. Yet only recently — in many countries — have the medical, public health and public policy communities begun to assess critically how best to respond to the inexorable rise in NCDs.

Thailand achieved unusually early success in reducing child mortality and infectious disease mortality more generally with one consequence being the aging of its population and concomitant rise in NCDs. Also unusually, Thailand invested early and substantially to create the analytic capacity to identify and develop approaches to NCD prevention and management. The Thai Health Ministry's Health Intervention and Technology Assessment Programs (HITAP), as well as closely associated efforts at Mahidol University, have provided world leadership in developing and applying techniques of economic evaluation to help ensure that public money spent on health buys the greatest possible reduction in premature mortality and morbidity. This timely volume — *Non-Communicable Disease Prevention: Best Buys, Wasted Buys and Contestable Buys* — brings to a global audience a distillation of much of HITAP's experience. An international editorial team was formed to match authors to topics. Then a broadly inclusive and iterative process of chapter development, described in Chapter 1, led to a volume that will become required reading for two important audiences: one concerned with implementation of strategies for NCD control and, significantly, the community of economists and others seeking an up-to-date account of how best to apply economic methods in practice.

Three important characteristics contribute to making this book an unusually informative resource. First, the volume results from an extensive international collaboration of individuals and institutions. This collaboration enriches the book's content and facilitates communication with diverse audiences. Second and closely related, the volume relies heavily on case studies to convey its main message — a total of fifty-eight case studies from thirty countries. The case studies ground the lessons of the book in operational experience and should prove of particular salience to NCD program managers, an audience the volume particularly tries to reach. Finally, this book develops and present a practical guide to the assessment of intervention attractiveness — the 'Systemic thinking for Evidence-based and Efficient Decision-making (SEED)' tool. SEED provides a valuable framework both for the book itself and for its application in practice.

It is not my purpose in this brief forword to overview this rich a volume. Nonetheless, I would like to touch on three points that resonated with my own experience working on the Disease Control Priorities (DCP) Project and, in particular, on issues that various iterations of DCP have had to deal with over many years.[1] One concerns the quality and transferability of evidence. A second persistent issue concerns economic evaluation when an intervention has significant non-health consequences (what the volume's authors call cross-sectoral intervention). Third, the volume's title points to consideration of Wasted Buys as well as Best Buys, a topic too often neglected in the literature. On each of these issues the authors provide valuable insights.

Two of the volume's chapters discuss evidence: one focuses on the synthesis of evidence of varying degrees of quality; and another on transferring findings from one setting or population to another and perhaps to very different settings or populations. The volume concurs in the general observation that randomized-controlled trials (RCTs) provide the highest quality evidence, but it is equally insistent in pointing out

---

1 Dean T. Jamison et al., *Disease Control Priorities: Improving Health and Reducing Poverty* (Washington, DC: World Bank, 2017), 3rd edition, IX.

that an RCT must be supplemented by judgement about transferability if the results are to be applied outside of the original setting. 'Hard' evidence can become soft very quickly and the DCP approach has been to acknowledge the ever-present need for informed judgement about the relevance and transferability of evidence. The explicit objective of the DCP's approach has been to balance concerns about accepting that an intervention is attractive when it is not — unfortunately the dominant concern of the medical community — with apprehension about rejecting an intervention that might be appropriate. The approach advocated in this book provides a welcome, systematic approach to facilitate judgement in this necessary search for balance. This approach can be applied equally to two other areas where judgement is required: evaluating the effect of a combined intervention (multi-drug approaches to secondary prevention of vascular disease, for example, when trials have been undertaken only on single-drug regimens); and deciding whether two different interventions (two health promotion campaigns or two anti-hypertensive drugs, for examples) can be viewed as essentially the same in terms of efficacy.

Reducing behavioral and environmental risk often involves action outside the health sector. Issuing and enforcing controls on air quality, for example, could result in significant reductions in mortality in many cities. Health ministries lack money and mandates to issue such regulations and, even if they did, there are likely to be significant benefits that derive from such investments that are unrelated to health. An economic evaluation of air quality regulation that relies on a standard incremental cost-effectiveness assessment — cost per death averted, say — will fail to capture all relevant benefits. On the other hand, an economic evaluation from the perspective of an energy ministry may simply neglect to consider health benefits. This book includes a thoughtful chapter on how to approach this problem within a cost-effectiveness framework. DCP authors assessing cross-sectoral intervention have tended either to report 'dashboards' of outcomes, without aggregation into a single figure of merit, or to use monetary metrics within a benefit-cost analysis (BCA) framework. I don't see an approach that is obviously best (although I lean toward BCAs). This book very much contributes to the thinking on this topic and national experience with the methods explained here will, over time, provide insight into what is practical and useful.

Separating economic evaluation from advocacy can prove difficult. Groups that work on immunization (or any other interventions you can name) often do so from a laudable commitment to the value of what they are doing. Likewise, because of their interest, these groups often commission or participate in economic evaluations. It requires no conscious bias to have results lean toward the favorable. Thus, this book's explicit argument for the importance of also considering Wasted Buys is very much to be welcomed. My own experience in DCP was that asking authors to identify interventions of low priority met with little success. Most DCP authors — there were important exceptions — simply avoided doing this. It appears that the authors of this book experienced similar problems. They report that of the fifty-eight case studies received, forty-seven were of Best Buys, seven were Contestable Buys and only four were Wasted Buys. This simply underscores this volume's contribution to generating sustained and serious consideration of what not to do (or to do only later). The inclusion of Wasted Buys in the title of the book and in the analysis sends a good message.

******

Analysts often neglect the political economy of implementation. One could argue that there is a natural division of labor between analysis and the politics of implementation (and in the past I have so argued). This book takes the perspective that considerations of political economy need inclusion from the outset. It is reasonable to predict that this explicit approach will combine with the book's analytic strength to give it enduring value.

Prof. Dean T. Jamison

Institute for Global Health Sciences
University of California, San Francisco

Acknowledgements

First, we would like to thank our funders for their generous support and for making our vision for this project a reality: the Prince Mahidol Award Foundation (PMAF), the Thai Health Promotion Foundation (THF) and the international Decision Support Initiative (iDSI).

The editors gratefully acknowledge the contribution of all the authors of this work, for without their diligence, commitment and expertise, this book would not have been possible. We specifically thank the following: Dr. Adam Elshaug (University of Sydney, Australia), Ms. Alia Luz (Health Intervention and Technology Assessment Program (HITAP), Thailand), Ms. Arisa Shichijo (Hitotsubashi University, Japan), Dr. David Kim (Tufts Medical Center, United States), Dr. Jesse Boardman Bump (Harvard University, United States), Dr. Kalipso Chalkidou (Center for Global Development in Europe, United Kingdom), Ms. Manushi Sharma (HITAP, Thailand), Dr. Melitta Zsuzsanna Jakab (World Health Organization, Spain), Dr. Peter Neumann (Tufts Medical Center, United States), Dr. Peter Smith (Imperial College London, United Kingdom), Ms. Rachel Bacon (Tufts Medical Center, United States), Dr. Ryota Nakamura (Hitotsubashi University, Japan), Ms. Sumithra Krishnamurthy Reddiar (Harvard University, United States), Dr. Tazeem Bhatia (Public Health England, United Kingdom), Dr. Thunyarat Anothaisintawee (Faculty of Medicine, Ramathibodi Hospital, Thailand) and Ms. Waranya Rattanavipapong (HITAP, Thailand). We would also like to thank the following individuals who have supported the writing of chapters. Thanks to Dr. Olaa Mohamed-Ahmed (Public Health England, United Kingdom) for their contribution to the appendices for Chapter 4 and thanks to Assistant Professor Kanokporn Sukhato, Dr. Kridsada

Chareonrungrueangchai and Dr. Keerati Wongkawinwoot (all from Ramathibodi Hospital, Thailand) for working on the study selection and data extraction of the umbrella review in Chapter 7.

We are especially grateful to Ms. Benjarin Santatiwongchai and Ms. Jirata Tienphati and rest of the HITAP communication team for their tireless support in the communication and presentation of this work. We also deeply appreciate all the efforts of the HITAP staff who have helped in the coordination and administration of the project.

Our external reviewers, whom we thank for their support in advancing our work, were: Dr. Amanda Glassman (Center for Global Development, United States), Dr. Shankar Prinja (PGIMER, India), Ms. Ursula Giedion (International Health Policy Consultant, Switzerland), Dr. Edwine Barasa (KEMRI-Wellcome Trust, Kenya), Dr. Arian Hatefi (University of California San Francisco, United States), Dr. Justin Parkhurst (London School of Economics, United Kingdom), Dr. Bundit Sornpaisarn (University of Toronto, Canada), Dr. Sara Bennett (Johns Hopkins Bloomberg School of Public Health, United States), Dr. Jeremy Addison Lauer (World Health Organization, Switzerland) and Ms. Priya Kanayson (NCD Alliance, United States).

Our thanks also to those listed below for reviewing our preliminary findings and also providing invaluable feedback:

Dr. Anita Jain (The BMJ, India)
Dr. Bundit Sornpaisarn (University of Toronto, Canada)
Dr. Chanuantong Tanasugarn (Mahidol University, Thailand)
Dr. Douglas Webb (United Nations Development Program, United States)
Ms. Emily Kobayashi (Clinton Health Access Initiative, United States)
Dr. Kanchan Mukherjee (Tata Institute of Social Sciences, India)
Dr. Karen Hofman (PRICELESS SA, South Africa)
Dr. Kelvin Tan (Ministry of Health, Singapore)
Ms. Milin Sakornsin (Thai Health Promotion Foundation, Thailand)
Dr. Myo Paing (World Health Organization, Myanmar)
Dr. Naomi Hamada (Ministry of Health and Medical Services, Fiji)
Mr. Pempa (Health Technology Assessment Program, Bhutan)
Ms. Saudamini Dabak (HITAP, Thailand)
Dr. Suchita Bhattacharyya (University of Liverpool, United Kingdom)
Dr. Sumudu Karunaratna (Ministry of Health, Sri Lanka)
Dr. Tea Collins (World Health Organization, Switzerland)

The authors of Chapter 2 and the project team gratefully acknowledge the contributions of their interviewees.

Finally, we owe a sincere thanks to the contributors who submitted case studies of their experiences with Best, Wasted and Contestable Buys in their local settings, in particular to Mr. Pempa, Dr. Rohan Jayasuriya, Dr. Sumudu Karunaratne and Dr. Amala de Silva, whose case studies were chosen as special features. We also acknowledge Dr. Koum Kanal, Dr. Karen Hofman, Mr. Gavin Surgey et al., Dr. Cristóbal Cuadrado and Ms. Frances Claire Onagan, whose case studies were discussed in the book. Thanks is also given to Ms. Aparna Ananthakrishnan from HITAP for proofreading this book.

Notes on Contributors

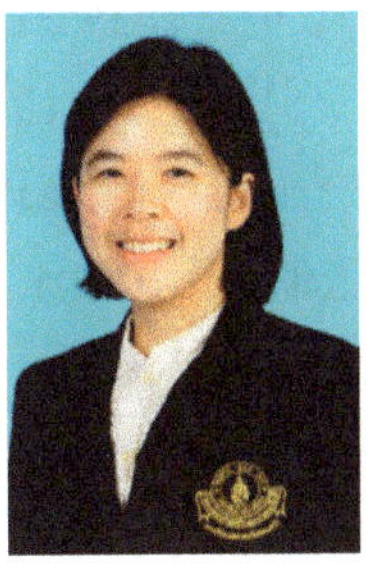

Thunyarat Anothaisintawee, MD., Ph.D., is a Family Physician. She holds a Ph.D. in Clinical Epidemiology and has worked as a faculty staff member at the Department of Family Medicine, Faculty of Medicine, Ramathibodi Hospital, Mahidol University, Thailand. She is an expert in systematic reviews and meta-analysis and published several papers about the association between sleep factors and risk of developing diabetes mellitus in international medical journals. Currently, she is conducting the Prediabetes cohort study in Thailand. This cohort aims to investigate the association between sleep factors, eating habits, level of physical activity, genetic factors and risk of developing diabetes mellitus and chronic kidney disease in prediabetes people in Thailand.

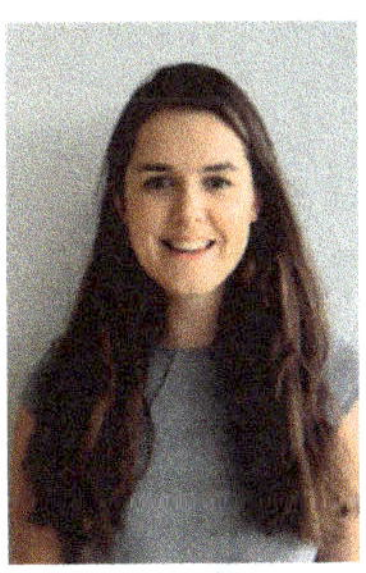

Rachel A. Archer, M.P.H., is a Project Associate at the Health Intervention and Technology Assessment Program (HITAP). Her work focuses on health system strengthening and supporting evidence-informed health policy making in low- and middle-income countries (LMICs). She is the focal point at HITAP for the Total Systems Effectiveness (TSE) project, an approach to strengthen vaccine decision-making in LMICs, and she currently leads the PMAC Commissioned Work project. Rachel has also supported capacity-building activities for Indonesia, Kenya and The Philippines. Rachel holds a Master's degree in Public Health from the University of Sheffield and a Bachelor of Arts in International Development from the University of Leeds. Whilst studying, she interned with various non-profit organizations across East and West Africa. For her Master's thesis, Rachel collaborated with a non-profit to investigate the trend towards teenage pregnancy in Luwero District, Uganda, through an intersectional framework. She was awarded the Carpenter Prize for Best Dissertation.

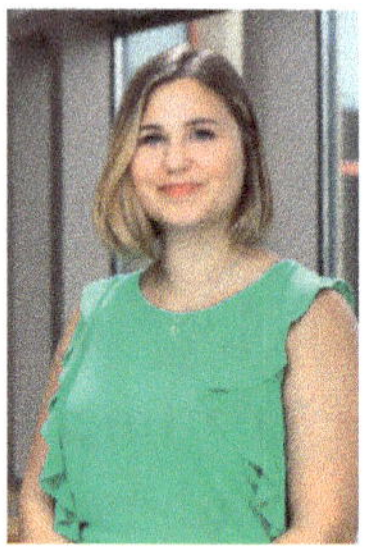

Rachel L. Bacon, M.P.H., is the Project Manager for global health initiatives at the Center for the Evaluation of Value and Risk in Health (CEVR) at the Institute for Clinical Research and Health Policy Studies (ICRHPS) at Tufts Medical Center. Rachel is a public health professional with knowledge and applied experience in global health, reproductive health, health economics, health systems strengthening, population health management, clinical business management and quality improvement. She has a strong cross-cultural work history, with consulting experience developed internationally within the United States, Sub-Saharan Africa, Europe and the Asia Pacific. She is a member of the Consortium of Universities for Global Health (CUGH), the International Society for Pharmacoeconomics and Outcomes Research (ISPOR) and the Institute for Health Care Improvement (IHI). She is also a trained labor and delivery birth doula with the Doula Organization of North America (DONA). Rachel holds a Master's of Public Health from Boston University and a Bachelor of Arts in Anthropology from the University of New Hampshire.

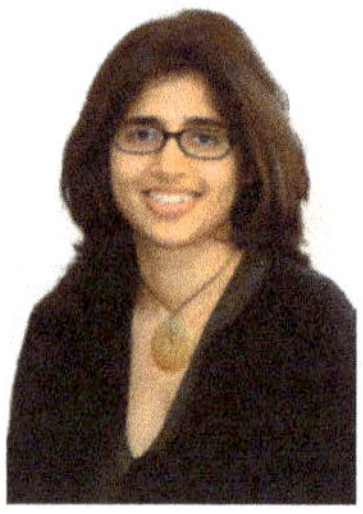

Tazeem Bhatia, MPhil., MD., MRCGP, is a Public Health and Primary Care physician with twenty years' experience of medical and public health practice in England, Myanmar, Afghanistan, Tajikistan and India. She has extensive expertise in the public health approach and tackling the wider determinants of health; community engagement and primary care; Universal Health Coverage (UHC) and models of social protection; and communicable and non-communicable disease (NCD) systems in high and low-income settings. She has conducted national level service and impact evaluations and sector wide health needs assessments, influencing senior leaders at a strategic level. She has worked in diverse environments and resource settings, from NGOs and think tanks, to Local Government, the NHS and UK Civil Service. Tazeem currently leads Public Health England's global engagement on non-communicable disease with a focus on obesity. This includes advocating through evidence generation for action on the upstream social determinants of health.

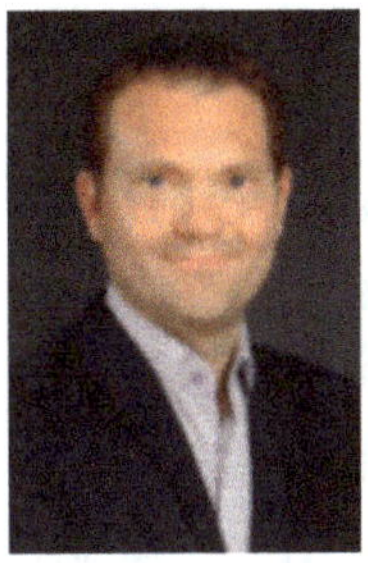

Jesse B. Bump, M.P.H, Ph.D., is Executive Director of the Takemi Program in International Health and Lecturer on Global Health Policy in the Department of Global Health and Population at the Harvard T. H. Chan School of Public Health. He leads the global health field of study in the Master of Public Health degree and teaches on the political economy of global health. His research focuses on the intellectual ecology of global health, examining the historical, political and economic forces that are among the most fundamental determinants of ill health, and the most significant contextual factors that shape institutions and the approaches they embrace. This work addresses major themes in global health history and in the political economy of global health to analyze these macro forces and develop strategies for navigating solutions within them.

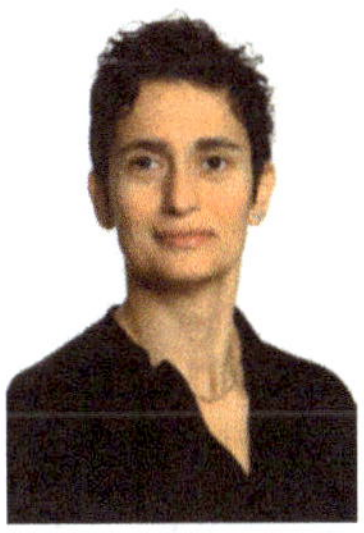

Kalipso Chalkidou, MD., Ph.D., is the Director of Global Health Policy and a Senior Fellow at the Center for Global Development, based in London and a Professor of Practice in Global Health at Imperial College London. Her work concentrates on helping governments build technical and institutional capacity for using evidence to inform health policy as they move towards Universal Healthcare Coverage. She is interested in how local information, local expertise and local institutions can drive scientific and legitimate healthcare resource allocation decisions. She has been involved in the Chinese rural health reforms and in national health reform projects in Colombia, Turkey and the Middle East, working with the World Bank, the Pan American Health Organization (PAHO), the Department for International Development (DFID) and the Inter-American Development Bank (IDB), as well as national governments. Between 2007 and 2008, she spent a year at the Johns Hopkins School of Public Health, as a Harkness fellow in Health Policy and Practice, studying how comparative effectiveness research can inform policy and US government drug pricing policies.

Kalipso led the establishment of NICE International, which she ran for eight years, and, more recently, of the international Decision Support Initiative (iDSI) which she directs and which is a multi-million, multi-country network working towards better health around the world through evidence-informed spending in healthcare in low to middle income countries. IDSI is funded by the Bill and Melinda Gates Foundation, the UK's Department for International Development and the Rockefeller Foundation and is currently involved in national reform projects in China, India, Vietnam, Ghana, Indonesia and South Africa working together with key organizations such as the Thai Health Intervention and Technology Assessment Program (HITAP), the US Center for Global Development and PRICELESS, at Wits University in South Africa.

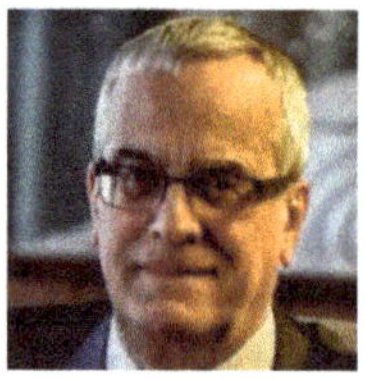

Anthony J. Culyer, Ph.D., is Emeritus Professor of Economics at the University of York (England), Senior Fellow at the Institute of Health Policy, Management and Evaluation at the University of Toronto (Canada) and Visiting Professor at Imperial College London. He is Chair of the Board of the international Decision Support Initiative (iDSI). He was the founding Organizer of the Health Economists' Study Group. For thirty-three years he was the founding Co-Editor, with Joe Newhouse at Harvard, of *Journal of Health Economics*. He was founding Vice Chair of the National Institute for Health and Care Excellence (NICE) until 2003. He is Editor-in-Chief of the online *Encyclopaedia of Health Economics*. For many years he was chair of the Department of Economics & Related Studies at York and, for six of them, was also deputy vice-chancellor. He has published widely, mostly in health economics.

He is a Founding Fellow of the Academy of Medical Sciences, an Honorary Fellow of the Royal College of Physicians of London and an Honorary Member of the Finnish Society for Health Economics (2013). He holds an honorary doctorate from the Stockholm School of Economics and is a Commander of the British Empire (CBE). He has been a member or chaired many policy committees and boards in the UK and Canada including authoring the 1994 reforms of NHS Research and Development and being a director of the Canadian Agency for Drugs and Technologies in Health (CADTH).

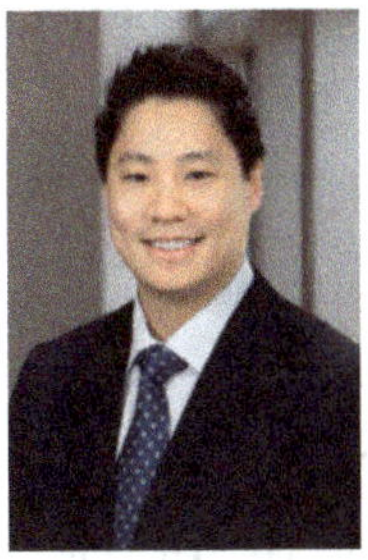

David D. Kim, Ph.D., is an Assistant Professor of Medicine at Tufts University School of Medicine and a Program Director of the CEA Registry at the Center for the Evaluation of Value and Risk in Health (CEVR) at the Institute for Clinical Research and Health Policy Studies (ICRHPS) at Tufts Medical Center. As a health economist, he has been passionate about generating the best available economic evidence to inform health care decisions and public health policies through mathematical modeling. His primary research focuses on developing disease simulation models; improving methodology in economic evaluation and research prioritization; understanding health and economic consequences of health policies; and examining access to and utilization of cost-effective health interventions. He has developed several disease models for hepatitis C, alcohol use disorders, diabetes, cancer and cardiovascular diseases. Also, as a lead author of the worked example included in the Second Edition of Cost-Effectiveness in Health and Medicine, he conducted a cost-effectiveness analysis to reflect the comprehensive guidelines and recommendations. David received his doctorate in Health Economics at the University of Washington and his Master's degree in Biostatistics from the University of Michigan.

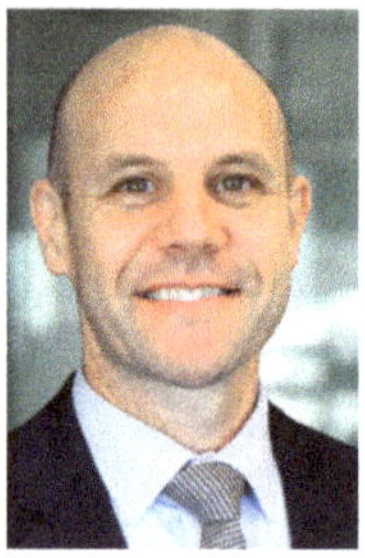

Adam Elshaug, M.P.H., Ph.D., is a researcher specializing in the calculation of low-value care and a policy advisor on approaches to reducing waste to optimize value in health care. He is Professor of Health Policy and Co-Director of the Menzies Centre for Health Policy (MCHP) at The University of Sydney, Australia and is a Visiting Fellow with the USC-Brookings Schaeffer Initiative for Health Policy at The Brookings Institution in the USA. Professor Elshaug has numerous committee and Board appointments, including as a Ministerial appointee to the (Australian) Medicare Benefits Schedule (MBS) Review Taskforce. This is a five-year process to review Australia's entire Medicare fee-for-service system utilizing Health Technology Assessment (HTA) principles and processes. Professor Elshaug was a 2010–2011 Commonwealth Fund Harkness Fellow based at the US Agency for Healthcare Research and Quality (AHRQ). From mid-2011 to mid-2013, he served as the National Health and Medical Research Council (NHMRC) Sidney Sax Fellow in Harvard Medical School's Department of Health Care Policy. He is the recipient of numerous research awards and has published over 130 technical reports and peer review articles with first-author publications in journals such as *The New England Journal of Medicine, BMJ* and *Journal of the American Medical Association*. Professor Elshaug was Co-Lead of 2017 'Right Care' Series of papers in *The Lancet*.

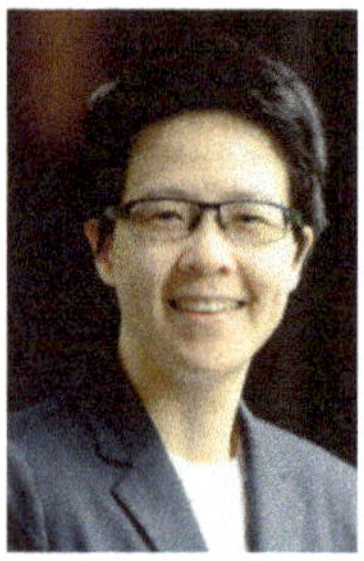

Wanrudee Isaranuwatchai, Ph.D., is a Senior Researcher at the Health Intervention and Technology Assessment Program (a part of the Ministry of Public Health) in Bangkok, Thailand, a Director at the Centre for Excellence in Economic Analysis Research of St. Michael's Hospital and a Senior Health Economist at the Canadian Centre for Applied Research in Cancer Control in Canada. She is also an Assistant Professor at the Institute of Health Policy, Management and Evaluation, University of Toronto. Her research focuses on how to apply economic evaluation in the real world setting as well as how to advance methods in economic evaluation. She has experience conducting economic evaluations using person-level data and decision modelling. She has collaborated with researchers and decision-makers in various areas to help communicate the value of health initiatives using economic evidence. Dr. Isaranuwatchai is dedicated to promoting the use of evidence in healthcare decision making.

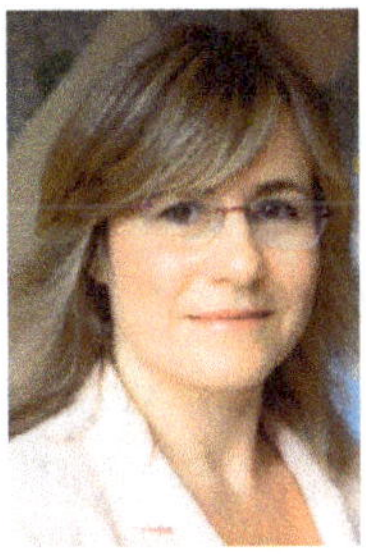

Melitta Jakab, M.Sc., Ph.D., is a senior health economist at the WHO Barcelona Office for Health Systems Strengthening. She has twenty years of experience in health system strengthening, health financing, policy analysis and education in global health. Her work includes advising WHO Member States on health financing policy design and implementation, in particular in Moldova, Kazakhstan, Kyrgyzstan, Tajikistan, Turkey, Ukraine and Uzbekistan. She has been leading a multidisciplinary work program on the Health System Response to NCDs. She has been co-director of the Barcelona Courses on Health Systems Strengthening and Health Financing. She is co-editor of Health Systems Respond to NCDs: Time for Ambition (Jakab, Farrington, Borgermans, Mantingh, WHO Regional Office for Europe 2018) and of Implementing Health Financing Reform: Lessons from Countries in Transition (Kutzin, Cashin and Jakab, European Observatory, 2010). She has a PhD from Harvard University and M.Sc. in Health Policy for the Harvard School of Public Health.

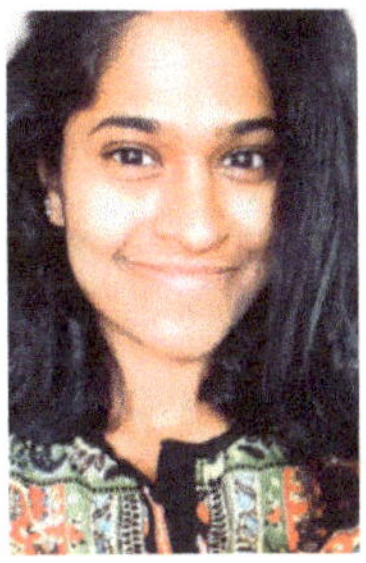

Sumithra Krishnamurthy, M.P.H., has a particular interest in the political and social implications of NCDs for vulnerable populations, with an emphasis on access to services. Sumithra holds an M.P.H. in Global Health from the Harvard T. H. Chan School of Public Health and received her Bachelor's degree in International Development from the University of Sussex in the UK. Her current research focuses on the political economy of NCDs from a global perspective. Sumithra has previously served at the United Nations Entity for Gender Equality and the Empowerment of Women (UN Women) as well as various civil society organizations in support of human rights and health in the UK, Mexico and Rwanda. She has also supported national health systems strengthening projects through consultancies in Mexico and Burkina Faso.

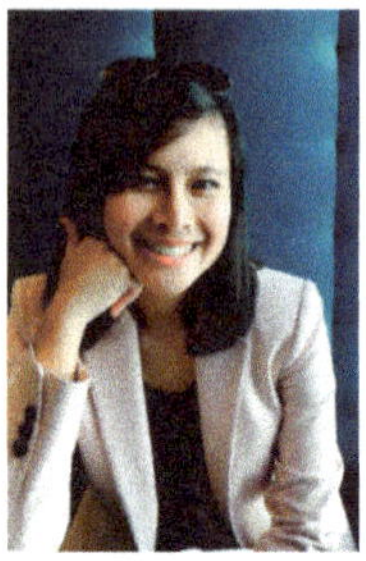

Alia Luz, M.Sc., works as a Project Associate with the management and research team of the international unit at Health Intervention and Technology Assessment Program (HITAP). She provides technical support in international and local economic evaluation projects, as well as administrative coordination for the organization's regional and country projects. Her portfolio of work includes management of HITAP projects in the Philippines, as well as the Guide to Economic Analysis and Research (GEAR) online resource. In 2018, she received her Masters of Science (M.Sc.) in Health Policy, Planning and Financing (HPPF) from both the London School of Hygiene and Tropical Medicine (LSHTM) and the London School of Economics (LSE). Alia graduated from Bryn Mawr College in 2013 with a degree in economics. Post-graduation, she worked in Liberia on renewable energy economics for a project funded by the United States Agency for International Development (USAID).

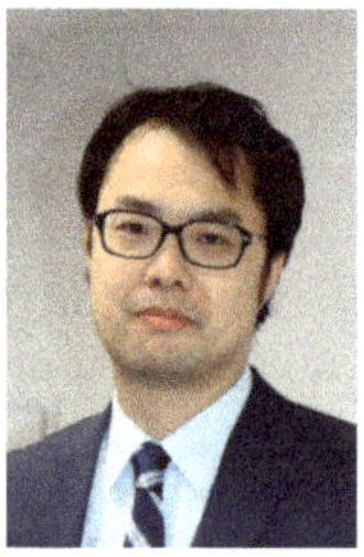

Ryota Nakamura, M.A., Ph.D., is an Associate Professor based in the Hitotsubashi Institute for Advanced Study (HIAS), Hitotsubashi University. He also serves as a Visiting Associate Professor at the Institute of Statistical Mathematics. He is an applied microeconomist specializing in health. He holds a B.A. and an M.A. in Economics from Kyoto University and a Ph.D. in Economics from the University of York in the UK. Prior to joining Hitotsubashi University in 2016, he held positions at the University of East Anglia and the University of York. His research interests include empirical and theoretical investigations of health-related behavior, as well as of healthcare systems to inform national and international public health policies, using a wide range of research methods including micro-econometric analysis of observational data e.g., impact evaluation), economic experiment, modelling and evidence synthesis.

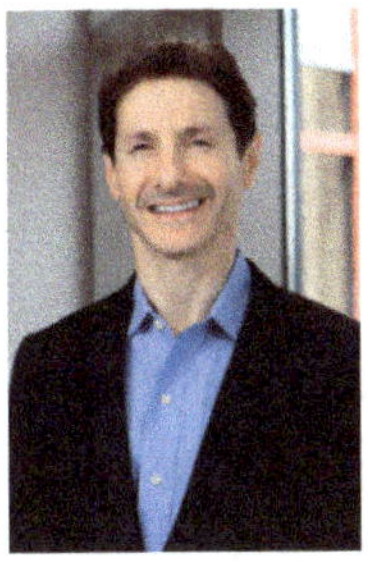

Peter J. Neumann, Sc.D., is Director of the Center for the Evaluation of Value and Risk in Health (CEVR) at the Institute for Clinical Research and Health Policy Studies at Tufts Medical Center and Professor of Medicine at Tufts University School of Medicine. He is the Founder and Director of the Cost-Effectiveness Analysis Registry. Dr. Neumann has written widely on clinical and economic evidence and on regulatory and reimbursement issues. He served as co-chair of the 2nd Panel on Cost-Effectiveness in Health and Medicine. He is the author or co-author of over 250 papers in medical literature, the author of *Using Cost-Effectiveness Analysis to Improve Health Care* (Oxford University Press, 2005) and co-editor of *Cost-Effectiveness in Health and Medicine*, 2nd Edition (Oxford University Press, 2016). Dr. Neumann has served as President of the International Society for Pharmacoeconomics and Outcomes Research (ISPOR). He is a member of the editorial advisory board of Health Affairs and the health policy advisory board for the Congressional Budget Office. He has held several policy positions in Washington, including Special Assistant to the Administrator at the Health Care Financing Administration. He received his doctorate in health policy and management from Harvard University.

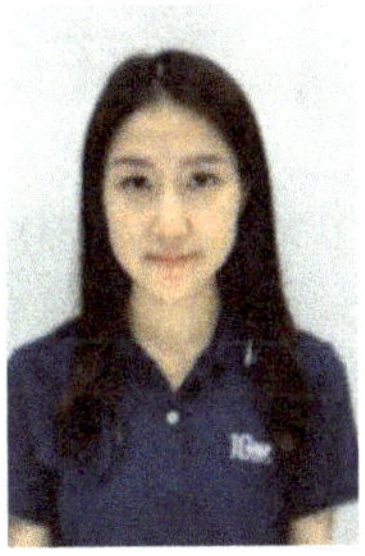

Waranya Rattanavipapong, M.Sc., joined Health Intervention and Technology Assessment Program (HITAP) in February 2010. She gained her Master's degree in Health Economics and Decision Modelling from the University of Sheffield in 2014. She has strong expertise in health economic evaluations and has been involved in several research projects to support the Thai government as well as the public agencies in Bhutan, Indonesia, India and Vietnam.

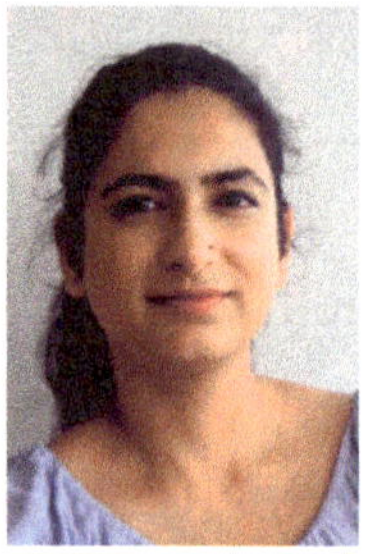

Manushi Sharma, M.B.A., is an International Cooperation Officer at the Health Intervention and Technology Assessment Program (HITAP). She is a pharmacist by training with a Master's in Business Management (M.B.A.). Previously, she worked with the Public Health Foundation of India with the health-economics and financing group. In the past, as a part of HITAP international unit (HIU), she has managed the iDSI Indonesia workstream. Currently, she is leading the monitoring and evaluation for all projects under HIU along with networking activities.

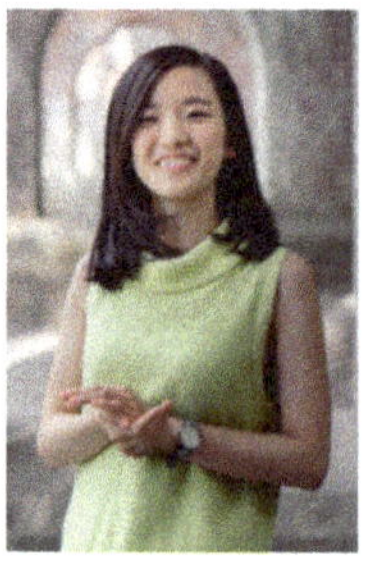

Arisa Shichijo, M.P.P., joined the project as a chapter team member. She received a B.A. in Law and Political science from Kyoto University and she is a second-year Master's student at the School of International and Public Policy Hitotsubashi University. Her main field of research is health economics with a special focus on the process of policymaking and implementations in health-related areas and empirical analysis to inform public health interventions. She also completed a one-year exchange at McGill University, with a focus on Health Policy. She is now a Research Assistant at the Hitotsubashi Institute for Advanced Study (HIAS).

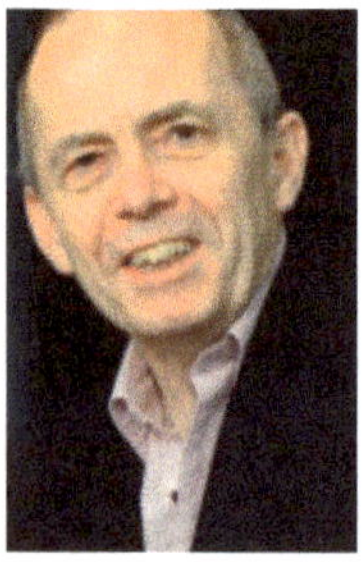

Peter C. Smith, Ph.D., is Emeritus Professor of Health Policy at Imperial College London and Honorary Professor of Health Economics, University of York. He is a mathematics graduate from the University of Oxford, with previous appointments at the University of Cambridge and the University of York, where he was Director of the Centre for Health Economics. His main research interest is in the economics of health, and his recent work has focused mainly on the financing and efficiency of health systems in low- and middle-income countries. Peter has published over 150 academic articles and twelve books, and has advised many governments and international agencies, including the World Health Organization, the

International Monetary Fund, the Global Fund, the World Bank, the European Commission and the Organization for Economic Cooperation and Development.

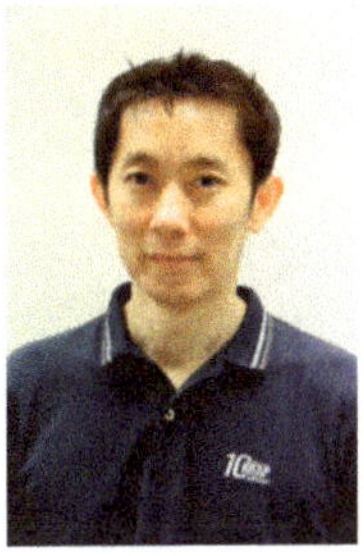

Yot Teerawattananon, MD., Ph.D., is the founding leader of the Health Intervention and Technology Assessment Program (HITAP), which is a semi-autonomous research institute of Thailand's Ministry of Public Health. The works of HITAP have been used to inform policy decisions regarding the adoption of medicines, medical devices, health promotion and disease prevention programmes under the Universal Health Coverage Scheme and the national pharmaceutical reimbursement list, the National List of Essential Medicines. Recently, he joins the National University of Singapore as a visiting professor at Saw Swee Hock School of Public Health as well as is the Executive Board of the international Decision Support Initiative (iDSI). He has published more than 140 peer-reviewed journal articles and provided technical support on HTA capacity building in Asia and Africa. He is also one of the founders of HTAsiaLink, a regional network comprising governmental health technology assessment agencies in the Asia and Pacific region.

1. Introduction

Wanrudee Isaranuwatchai, Rachel A. Archer and Anthony J. Culyer

1.1 Non-Communicable Disease

Non-communicable diseases (NCDs) are the leading cause of death worldwide and contribute to over 73% of all deaths annually.[1] Each day, NCDs cause more than 100,000 deaths; 80% of which occur in low- and middle-income countries (LMICs).[2] Over the last 30 years, NCDs have replaced communicable diseases (CDs) as the cause of greatest health burden.[3] This trend is evident in the risk factors for NCDs. According to the World Health Organization (WHO), obesity has tripled since 1975;[4] while the International Diabetes Federation estimates that the global prevalence of diabetes, 8.8% in 2017, will increase by 48% by 2045, with an additional 204 million people living with diabetes.[5] Much of this burden could be completely avoided because NCDs are largely preventable.[6] Approximately 40% of all cancers and three-quarters

1 Our World In Data, *What Do People Die From?*, 2018, https://ourworldindata.org/what-does-the-world-die-from

2 World Health Organization, *Non-communicable Diseases,* 2018, https://www.who.int/news-room/fact-sheets/detail/noncommunicable-diseases

3 Institute for Health Metrics and Evaluation, *Global Burden of Disease (GBD)*, 2019, http://www.healthdata.org/gbd

4 World Health Organization Newsroom, *Obesity and Overweight: Key Facts*, 2018, https://www.who.int/en/news-room/fact-sheets/detail/obesity-and-overweight

5 International Diabetes Federation, *IDF Diabetes Atlas — 8th Edition*, 2017, https://diabetesatlas.org/resources/2017-atlas.html

6 World Health Organization, *10 Facts on Non-communicable Diseases,* 2019, https://www.who.int/features/factfiles/noncommunicable_diseases/facts/en/index4.html

 https://doi.org/10.11647/OBP.0195.01

of the incidence of heart disease, stroke and type 2 diabetes could be prevented by addressing tobacco use, unhealthy diet, physical inactivity and harmful use of alcohol. A great deal of technical knowledge exists about how to prevent and manage NCDs, such as the WHO Package of Essential NCD interventions (WHO PEN),[7] the SHAKE[8] (the technical package for salt reduction) and HEARTS[9] (the technical package for cardiovascular disease management in primary health care) packages.

In addition to the NCD burden,[10] there is an increasing demand on governments to address the health needs arising from NCDs through universal health coverage (UHC) policies, a direction that has been endorsed by the World Health Assembly[11] and the United Nations General Assembly.[12] NCDs are the result of various factors, for example genetic, physiological, and environmental and behavioral[13] individually or in combination. They frequently require a collective response. They are not contagious, unlike communicable or infectious diseases, which can be spread, directly or indirectly, from one person to another.[14] CDs, accidents and injuries also often need collective actions (such as mass vaccination or health and safety legislation) for

---

7 World Health Organization, *Tools for Implementing WHO PEN (Package of Essential Non-communicable Disease Interventions)*, 2019, https://www.who.int/ncds/management/pen_tools/en/

8 World Health Organization, *The SHAKE Technical Package for Salt Reduction*, 2016, https://apps.who.int/iris/bitstream/handle/10665/250135/9789241511346-eng.pdf?sequence=1

9 World Health Organization, *Hearts: Technical Package for Cardiovascular Disease Management in Primary Health Care.*, 2016, https://apps.who.int/iris/bitstream/handle/10665/252661/9789241511377-eng.pdf?sequence=1

10 David E. Bloom et al., *From Burden to 'Best Buys': Reducing the Economic Impact of Non-Communicable Diseases in Low-and Middle-Income Countries* (Geneva, 2011), http://apps.who.int/medicinedocs/documents/s18804en/s18804en.pdf; David E. Bloom et al., *The Global Economic Burden of Non-communicable Diseases, World Economic Forum: World Economic Forum and the Harvard School of Public Health* (Geneva, 2011).

11 World Health Organization, *World Health Assembly Resolution WHA67.23: Health Intervention and Technology Assessment in Support of Universal Health Coverage* (World Health Organization, 2014), http://apps.who.int/medicinedocs/en/m/abstract/Js21463en/

12 United Nations General Assembly, *United Nations General Assembly Resolution A/67/L.36: Global Health and Foreign Policy* (United Nations, 2012), https://documents-dds-ny.un.org/doc/UNDOC/LTD/N12/630/51/PDF/N1263051.pdf?OpenElement

13 World Health Organization, *'Non-communicable Diseases: Key Facts 2018'*, 2019, http://www.who.int/news-room/fact-sheets/detail/non-communicable-diseases

14 Mauricio L. Barreto et al., 'Infectious Diseases Epidemiology', *Journal of Epidemiology and Community Health*, 60 (2006), 192–95, http://dx.doi.org/10.1136/jech.2003.011593

effective treatment but can also be treated effectively on an individual basis. There are noticeable patterns in prevalence and mortality between CDs and NCDs. Figures 1.1 and 1.2 show the prevalence and mortality of CDs and NCDs in high-income countries (HICs), LMICs and around the globe.[15] CDs are prevalent (~70%) in HICs compared to ~45% in LMICs (Fig. 1.1). NCDs are more prevalent in LMICs (~55%) compared to HICs (~30%). From the 37 years of data examined for Global Burden of Disease Study 2016, NCDs now dominate premature death.[16] Over 80% of the world's premature deaths are attributable to NCDs in LMICs.[17] The probability of premature death from NCDs is almost four times higher in LMICs compared to HICs.[18]

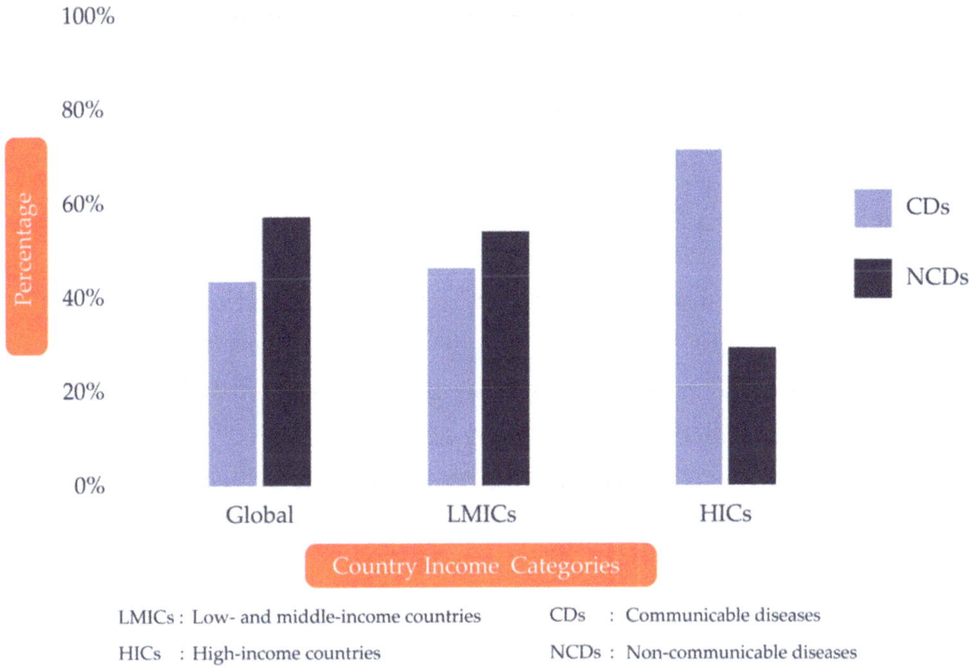

Fig. 1.1 Prevalence of CDs and NCDs by World Bank country income categories.[19]

15 Institute for Health Metrics and Evaluation, *Global Health Data Exchange*, 2016, http://ghdx.healthdata.org/

16 Ibid.

17 UN Interagency Task Force on NCDs, *Working Together for Health and Development: Prevention and Control of Non-Communicable Diseases*, 2017, https://www.who.int/ncds/un-task-force/working-together-adaptation.pdf?ua=1

18 Ibid.

19 World Health Organization, *10 Facts on Non-communicable Diseases*.

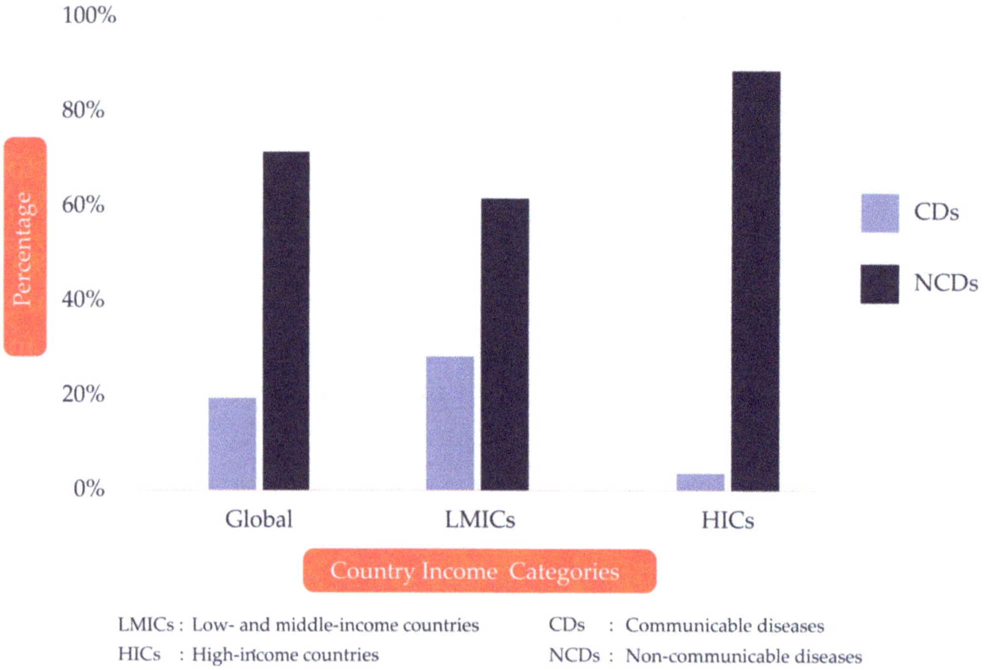

Fig. 1.2 Deaths from CDs and NCDs by World Bank country income categories.[20]

NCDs represent a significant burden through both an epidemiological and an economic lens.[21] They affect everyone regardless of sex and age.[22] The four main NCDs are cardiovascular disease, chronic respiratory disease, cancer and diabetes, which account for over 80% of NCDs deaths.[23] A macroeconomic simulation model suggested a cumulative loss of USD $47 trillion over the next 2 decades due to NCDs.[24] The Disease Control Priorities 3rd edition (DCP3) estimated that the number of deaths averted through prevention in LMICs could be between 2 to 4.2 million by 2030.[25] Additionally, mental health problems are the leading

20 Ibid.

21 Catherine P. Benziger et al., 'The Global Burden of Disease Study and the Preventable Burden of NCD', *Global Heart*, 11.4 (2016), 393–97, https://doi.org/10.1016/j.gheart.2016.10.024

22 World Health Organization, '10 Facts on Non-communicable Diseases', https://www.who.int/features/factfiles/non-communicable_diseases/facts/en/index4.html

23 World Health Organization, 'Non-communicable Diseases: Key Facts 2018', 2019, http://www.who.int/news-room/fact-sheets/detail/non-communicable-diseases

24 Bloom et al., *The Global Economic Burden of Non-communicable Diseases, World Economic Forum: World Economic Forum and the Harvard School of Public Health*

25 Dean T. Jamison et al., 'Universal Health Coverage and Intersectoral Action for Health: Key Messages from Disease Control Priorities', *The Lancet*, 11.4 (2018), 1108–20, https://doi.org/10.1016/S0140-6736(17)32906-9

cause of disability around the world.[26] For example, approximately 800,000 people commit suicide every year and about 75% of those occur in LMICs.[27] Mental health problems represent risk factors for other diseases such as cardiovascular diseases and diabetes including unintentional and intentional injury. There is significant inequity in the support (e.g., health services) for mental health around the world.

In an ideal world, it would be easy to prioritize interventions and allocate resources to have the maximum impact on health and its fair distribution, while simultaneously minimizing the risk to families of serious financial hardship from out-of-pocket payments. These are generally seen as the main concerns of cost-effectiveness analysis. Systems are, however, faced with a diversity of investment options, inescapable limits on resources, evidence that is at best sporadic, many other political, financial and social constraints, and a host of other additional[28] considerations; all of which make identifying good value-for-money interventions challenging. The question naturally arises: why have we, the global community, not been more successful at reducing this NCD burden? Does a universal problem not have a universal solution? Is resource scarcity the fundamental culprit? Is cost-effectiveness really the answer? Are there better ways of using the resources that countries already have? Do countries have the essential human capital required to develop and roll out the right policies? Are there higher priorities for public spending against which the NCDs simply cannot compete? We try to answer these questions and make some suggestions for future actions in this book.

1.2 Best, Wasted and Contestable Buys

One response by the WHO to the NCD crisis was the idea of 'Best Buys'. WHO defines Best Buys almost solely by their cost-effectiveness, that is, interventions which achieve best value for money in comparison to all comparators.[29] More precisely, Best Buys for LMICs are

26 World Health Organization, *10 Factors on Mental Health*, 2019, https://www.who.int/features/factfiles/mental_health/mental_health_facts/en/index1.html

27 Ibid.

28 See Chapter 4.

29 Bloom et al., *From Burden to 'Best Buys': Reducing the Economic Impact of Non-Communicable Diseases in Low-and Middle-Income Countries.*

interventions with an incremental cost-effectiveness ratio (ICER) under 100 International United States dollars per disability-adjusted life-year (DALY) averted.[30]

Some Wasted Buys are easy to define: they are interventions that have no beneficial effect. Others are slightly harder to specify, for they are interventions that do have a beneficial effect (with NCDs, the effect almost always lies in the more distant future) but ones that require too great a sacrifice of resources. That is, those resources would have a more beneficial effect used elsewhere on other health interventions or elsewhere in the economy. In other words, their opportunity cost is too high.

We suggest the addition of the category 'Contestable Buys' when there are suggestions that an intervention and its associated attributes may be a Best Buy but there is no direct evidence of cost-effectiveness in the local setting in which the intervention might be implemented. Thus, interventions in the WHO's Best Buys list may be better classed as Contestable Buys if there is no demonstrative evidence of cost-effectiveness for the particular setting in question. The main distinction between Best and Contestable Buys is thus the availability of context-specific evidence.

1.3 Definitions and Central Ideas

Box 1.1 contains the definitions of central ideas that are used throughout the book. The reader will find these definitions to vary slightly from the many that lie elsewhere in the literature, though we are confident that any differences are minor and more questions of emphasis than of substance. We — all the authors here represented — have sought to be consistent in the way we have used these terms.

We refer frequently to 'interventions'. This word is intended as an all-embracing term to capture a package of care over a relevant time period as applied to a particular condition or combination of morbidities. It may be restorative, maintenance or preventive. It may be provided in part from a health service program and partly from another like childcare or primary education. This is especially significant in the field of NCDs, with which

30 The DALY is one of several frequently met measures of the effectiveness of health care interventions. It stands for 'Disability-Adjusted Life-Year' where the Life-Year is a year of life gained and an adjustment is then made for the quality of life in terms of presence or absence of disabilities. A measure of health *gain* is therefore a DALY *averted*.

this book is concerned. An intervention should not be seen as merely the purchase and use of a medicine, or any other single input, but rather as the planned or usual combination of human and physical resources required for the delivery of a service at a chosen standard. Some of these inputs may not be what we customarily think of as 'healthcare'.

A critical starting point in determining the value of an intervention is its cost-effectiveness — if an analysis establishes empirical evidence of cost-effectiveness in the context of the location in which it is intended to be used, the intervention will be categorized as a 'Best Buy'. If it establishes empirical evidence of its cost inefficiency, it will essentially be categorized as a 'Wasted Buy' or if it confers very little effectiveness, that is, the costs are not proportional to effectiveness, then it will again be categorized as a Wasted Buy.

Box 1.1 Definitions of Basic Terminology Used in Economic Evaluation

Economic evaluation is the comparative analysis of two or more alternatives in terms of their costs and outcomes. There are different types of economic evaluation, namely cost-benefit analysis, cost-minimization analysis, cost-utility analysis and cost-effectiveness analysis. They differ primarily in the measurement of consequences or outcome; however, each approach entails value judgements that should be explicitly considered in terms of their appropriateness in the decision context.

Cost-effectiveness analysis (CEA) is a form of economic evaluation that uses monetary units to measure/value costs and (usually) a single effect of interest that is common to the alternatives in consideration. The effect is measured in terms of clinical natural units (e.g., life-years gained). Often, cost-effectiveness analyses are interchangeable with cost-utility analysis that uses generic outcome measures such as the quality-adjusted life-year (QALY) or disability-adjusted life- year (DALY) instead of clinical natural effects. The advantage of the cost-utility analysis approach over cost-effectiveness analysis is that the former allows comparison of value in health investment between different health problems such as diabetes and mental health.

Disability-adjusted life-year (DALY) is a measure of overall disease burden, expressed as the total number of years of life lost due to ill-health, disability, or premature death. One DALY is equal to one year of healthy life lost.

Quality-adjusted life-year (QALY) is a measure of the state of health of a person or group, which is a function of the length and quality of life. One QALY is equal to one year of life in perfect health.

Incremental cost-effectiveness ratio (ICER) is calculated as the difference in cost between two possible interventions, divided by the difference in their outcomes. It is a standard measure representing marginal cost per marginal benefit from health investment.

Health Technology Assessment (HTA) is a form of evaluation that includes CEA but goes beyond its categories by including non-financial constraints and local environmental, organizational, social and political factors that may affect the costliness, effectiveness and feasibility of interventions.

Sources: adapted from Drummond et al., 2015 and Briggs et al., 2006.[31]

1.4 The Cost-Effectiveness Plane

These ideas are illustrated by what is called a Cost-Effectiveness Plane. In Fig. 1.3, the health effects of an intervention are measured in terms of lives saved, QALYs, DALYs averted, or other suitable indicators on the horizontal axis (positive effects to the right and negative ones to the left). Its relative costliness is shown by the vertical axis. A comparator intervention can be understood to be at the origin where the two axes cross, so the health gain and the cost are both relative to a comparator. The distances along the axes measure the difference between the intervention under investigation and the comparator. The slope of the dashed line labelled 'threshold' indicates the willingness of the payer (usually an insurer or the government) to pay for additional health

31 Michael F Drummond et al., *Methods for the Economic Evaluation of Health Care Programmes* (Oxford: Oxford University Press, 2015); Andrew Briggs, Mark Sculpher and Karl Claxton, *Decision Modelling for Health Economic Evaluation* (Oxford: Oxford University Press, 2006).

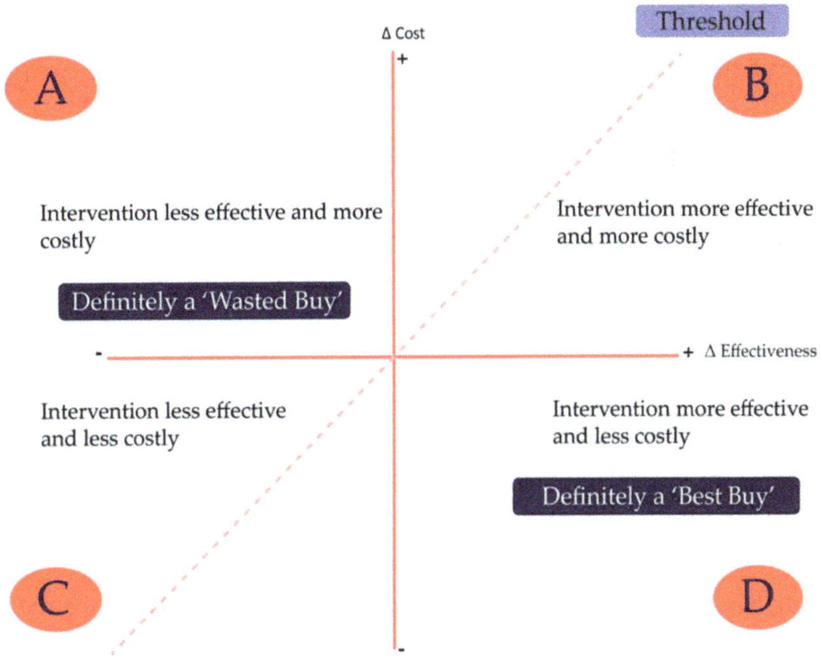

Fig. 1.3 Cost-effectiveness plane.

(ΔC/ΔE): the ICER. This threshold is also known as the cost-effectiveness threshold or willingness-to-pay (WTP) threshold and is expected to be different for each country setting.[32] That being so, what is regarded as cost-effective will also differ according to country.

The area lying in quadrant D clearly identifies a Best Buy — the intervention is both more effective and less costly than a relevant comparator. The area lying in quadrant A is clearly a Wasted Buy. D and A are areas in which an intervention dominates or is dominated by the comparator in terms of cost-effectiveness and its position relative to the threshold. This analysis is a development of the approach taken by the Institute of Medicine's (IOM) famous book *Crossing the Quality Chasm*.[33] In discussing efficiency as one of the six specific aims for improvement in health care, the book asserts that 'the opposite of efficiency is waste, the use of resources without benefit to the patients a system is intended to help'.[34]

32 Hilary F. Ryder et al., 'Decision Analysis and Cost-Effectiveness Analysis', *Seminars in Spine Surgery*, 21.4 (2009), 216–22, https://doi.org/10.1053/j.semss.2009.08.003

33 Institute of Medicine (U.S.), *Committee on Quality of Health Care in America: Crossing the Quality Chasm: A New Health System for the 21st Century* (Washington, DC: National Academy Press, 2001).

34 Jaqueline Zinn and Ann Barry Flood, 'Commentary: Slack Resources in Health Care Organizations-Fat to Be Trimmed or Muscle to Be Exercised?', *Health Services Research*, 44.3 (2009), 812–20, https://doi.org/10.1111/j.1475-6773.2009.00970.x

What of areas B and C? An intervention falling in B could be either a Best Buy or a Wasted Buy. In quadrant B, the intervention is more expensive but it is also more effective, so the question become whether the additional effectiveness is 'worth' the additional expense. Here, the dashed line comes into play because cost-effectiveness will depend on the maximum amount the payer is willing to spend for additional health outcomes. When the intervention is located above the dashed line, the additional or incremental cost (ΔC) exceeds the payer's willingness to pay for the additional or incremental health (ΔE), and the intervention will be judged to be cost-ineffective by the payer and therefore a Wasted Buy. Conversely, an intervention falling below the threshold line will be deemed cost-effective and therefore a Best Buy.

Quadrant C brings up some counter-intuitive possibilities. In this quadrant, the intervention is definitely less effective than the comparator. However, it is also less costly. Again, whether it would be a Wasted Buy depends on whether the cost savings of using it sufficiently compensate for using this intervention rather than its more effective comparator. How can this be? Only if the cost savings, if realized, can be used to generate more health elsewhere. In quadrant B, the threshold line indicates the maximum willingness of the payer to pay for additional units of health. In quadrant C, the line indicates the minimum the payer is willing to accept to forgo a marginal health benefit. If the threshold genuinely indicates the payer's judgment of value, then an intervention located below the dashed line will indicate a larger cost saving than the minimum indicated as acceptable by the dashed line. Paradoxically, then, a less effective intervention need not be a Wasted Buy — as long as it is also sufficiently cheaper than the comparator it will replace. It may even be a Best Buy!

Various techniques have been used to define thresholds. The three most popular methods[35] are:

- deriving the threshold from previous decisions or other jurisdictions,
- the willingness to pay of the payer ('demand-side method'), or
- value of displaced services ('supply-side method').

35 Anthony J. Culyer, 'Cost-Effectiveness Thresholds in Health Care: A Bookshelf Guide to Their Meaning and Use', *Health Economics, Policy and Law,* 11.4 (2016), 415–32, https://doi.org/10.1017/s1744133116000049

The latter two have gained popularity and are the most cited approaches. However, each has limitations. The demand-side approach requires the society's or the government's willingness to pay (WTP) for healthcare to determine the threshold that would guide expenditures from the healthcare budget accordingly. In most cases, society's willingness to pay will be set explicitly or implicitly by the government. The chosen threshold will inevitably be controversial, so the methods used to determine it should be well-founded, clear and transparent. Where experts are consulted, they should be of appropriate distinction and independence. Calculating an aggregate social willingness to pay by asking citizens is also fraught with difficulties and can be controversial. The WHO previously adopted the approach of the first bullet in the list above. It generated a global threshold ratio taking the form that interventions costing less than three times the average per capita income per disability-adjusted life-years (DALY) averted were considered to be cost-effective and those exceeding this level were considered to be cost-ineffective.[36] Subsequently, there was an updated suggestion that the threshold could be between one to three Gross Domestic Product (GDP) per capita.[37] This approach in both cases implicitly assumed that there is fixed relationship between GDP and the appropriate magnitude of expenditure on healthcare, despite this being a policy decision that can legitimately vary depending on local priorities. Context and additional considerations[38] are matters that should be considered prior to the implementation of any threshold. A global threshold for all countries is an average (which may be generally too high or too low) but will rarely exactly fit the conditions in any particular country and may lead countries into committing themselves to merely Contestable Buys or, worse, to Wasted Buys.[39]

The threshold, though potentially useful, is not itself a decision rule. It is only a guide. There may be circumstances under which a country

36 Tessa-Tan-Torres Edejer et al., 'Making Choices in Health: WHO Guide to Cost-Effectiveness Analysis', (Geneva: World Health Organization, 2003), https://www.who.int/choice/publications/p_2003_generalised_cea.pdf

37 World Health Organization, *World Health Organization, Cost-Effectiveness Thresholds*, 2012, http://www.who.int/choice/costs/CER_thresholds/en/index.html

38 See Chapter 4.

39 Melanie Y. Bertram et al., 'Cost-Effectiveness Thresholds: Pros and Cons', *Bulletin of the World Health Organization*, 94.12 (2016), 925–30, https://doi.org/10.2471/blt.15.164418

may rationally choose to admit interventions that have ICERs above the threshold or reject some that lie below it. For analyses that try to take account of factors other than cost-effectiveness in deciding whether an intervention is a Best Buy, one may turn to Health Technology Assessment (HTA).

Cost-saving and cost-effectiveness are not synonyms. Depending on the context, it is possible, especially in a highly resource-constrained setting, that a less expensive and slightly less effective strategy is preferable, and vice-versa; interventions that are expensive may be cost-effective if they result in significant health outcomes and the cost-effectiveness threshold is sufficiently high.

These, then, are the basic ideas around which this book is built. What initially seems clear, and even obvious, turns out to be complex, controversial and may require the tools of Health Technology Appraisal (HTA) rather than those of CEA alone.

1.5 The Story of This Book

The Prince Mahidol Award Conference (PMAC) was first convened in 2007 and has continued annually since. This global health forum honors the memory of Prince Mahidol of Songkla, who dedicated his life's work to advancing public health and medical practice in Thailand and is respectfully regarded as the Father of Modern Medicine and Public Health of Thailand. Further information about PMAC is available via this link: https://pmaconference.mahidol.ac.th/site.

At a preparatory meeting for PMAC 2019, the slow progress towards global NCD targets was a major topic for discussion, particularly how the inadequate implementation of effective NCD prevention interventions contributes to this failure. Dr. Yot Teerawattananon, the founding leader of the Health Intervention and Technology Assessment Program (HITAP), emphasized that inefficiency in healthcare hinders progress. Working in collaboration with the International Decision Support Initiative (iDSI) (https://www.idsihealth.org/), which is a network of priority-setting organizations, HITAP has found that low-value health interventions are a significant contributor to wasteful spending in health.

With the financial support from PMAC, the Thai Health Promotion Foundation and iDSI, and in collaboration with several other global partners, HITAP developed a concept note for a practical guide to assist program managers in identifying good solutions (Best Buys) and avoid poor choices (Wasted Buys) for the prevention of NCDs. The concept note was accepted by the PMAC Scientific Committee in Tokyo in May 2018 and the initiative 'Non-Communicable Disease Prevention: Best Buys, Wasted Buys and Contestable Buys' was born.

1.6 The Project and Its Output

The project brought together experts from various disciplines in health economics, health policy, political economy, public health practice and NCDs. HITAP, which served as the project's secretariat, invited various organizations and individuals in its wider network to join the authorship team. In total, we have 20 authors from 14 organizations in 8 countries. Authors were assigned a chapter from the concept note according to their expertise; some chapters were co-authored by members of several organizations. The output was always conceived as something much more than a book. Our findings were to be disseminated through knowledge translation materials such as videos, blogs, animations and interactive seminars. The project aimed to create an evidence package to support health program managers when thinking about NCD prevention. The evidence package as finalized includes the printed book, the online book, online appendices (which include further details on the project, such as additional descriptions on methods), interview clips with policy-makers on the topic of NCD prevention, and a website.[40] More details can be found on the project website: https://www.buyitbestncd.health.

1.7 The Project Journey

An initial in-person meeting was held in August 2018 for 12 members of the project team. This meeting enabled the project team members to meet

40 The printed, digital and online editions of this book, together with the online appendices, can be found on the Open Book Publishers website, https://www.openbookpublishers.com/product/1113

one another and enabled the authors to present and receive comments on the outlines they had developed. Additionally, discussions prompted modifications to the form and structure of the book.

It was recognized that the work needed to be relevant to the target audience of NCD managers, that it should be written in comprehensible language and that it should draw whenever possible on managers' perceptions and experience. HITAP subsequently put out a call for LMIC-focused case studies on experiences of Best Buys, Wasted Buys or Contestable Buys in the prevention of NCDs. The call was circulated through various channels including: PMAC, iDSI, HTAsiaLink and WHO. In total, 58 case studies were received from thirty countries (https://www.buyitbestncd.health/about). Out of the fifty-eight cases submitted, forty-seven case studies that were deemed relevant were analyzed (see Chapter 4 on Best Buys).

A second, two-day, in-person meeting was convened in November 2019 with chapter leads, the editorial team, project organizers and observers. The preliminary drafts of the findings for each chapter were circulated with authors beforehand and systematically discussed. The concept note originally had the title *Best Buys, Wasted Buys and 'Do-It-Yourselves' (DIYs) in NCD Prevention*. The DIY term was dropped after much discussion, mainly because of its apparent endorsement of an individualistic approach to NCDs, and was replaced by 'Contestable Buys' to cover the many cases where Best and Wasted Buys could not be identified unambiguously.

Our initial ideas and some draft chapters were presented in January 2019 at PMAC 2019 (http://pmac2019.com/site) through two side-meetings and one main parallel session. The first side-meeting took the form of a closed meeting where eighteen external reviewers commented on the work to date. A second side-meeting was convened privately for authors to discuss how best to move forward following the feedback received in the previous side-meeting. This discussion resulted in some changes to the proposed content structure of the book and a commitment as far as possible to draw on real-world cases to illustrate points of principle and their practical application. A main parallel session at PMAC 2019 was open to the entire conference. Lead authors presented their chapters for five minutes followed by interactive questions and answers. This session was the best attended parallel session at PMAC 2019 and provided the basis for the final shape and content of the book.

After further draft revisions and editing, chapters and book were sent to ten experts for external review: each of the eight main chapters were assigned a reviewer, and two reviewers were entrusted with evaluating the book as a whole. After further revisions, the chapters were shared with the editorial team for final edits.

1.8 Target Audience

This book is written mainly with individuals who coordinate and/or have decision-making authority over NCD programs in mind. While their official job titles vary, we used the term 'NCD program managers' to encompass chronic disease or NCD managers, policy officers, project managers, scheme managers, implementers and evaluators operating in (non-)governmental organizations. Some of the common characteristics of the job roles and the managers' working environments are as follows. They:

- work in (non-)governmental 'NCD units' or 'sub units' dedicated to one or more of the main diseases (cardiovascular disease, diabetes, chronic lung disease, cancers and mental health) under the NCD umbrella, or to NCD risk factors;
- implement NCD health plans to the community;
- operate at the national, provincial, district or local level; and/or
- work on the integration of NCDs into existing service delivery platforms.

The target audience of this book thus consists of individuals who work in spheres of implementation. The work is, however, also intended to aid NCD champions, policy advocates and educators who spearhead the movement for increased visibility of NCDs and a reduction in the occurrence of these diseases.

2. Non-Communicable Diseases, NCD Program Managers and the Politics of Progress

Sumithra Krishnamurthy Reddiar and Jesse B. Bump

2.1 Background

Non-communicable diseases (NCDs) are a defining problem of the twenty-first century,[1] with an estimated economic loss of 7 trillion US dollars (USD) and counting to low- and middle-income countries (LMICs) between 2011 and 2025.[2] By 2020, NCDs are expected to cause seven out of every ten deaths in developing countries.[3] This challenge raises many questions, including how to raise the priority of NCDs on national policy agendas, augment capacities and identify resources to overcome it. Over the last decade, international agreements and three high-level meetings on NCDs held by the United Nations (UN) General Assembly (in 2011, 2014 and 2018)[4] have outlined the tolls NCDs

1 Sara Glasgow and Ted Schrecker, 'The Double Burden of Neoliberalism? Non-communicable Disease Policies and the Global Political Economy of Risk', *Health and Place*, 39 (2016), 204–11, https://doi.org/10.1016/j.healthplace.2016.04.003

2 World Health Organization and United Nations Development Programme, *What Legislators Need to Know: Non-communicable Diseases*, 2018, https://www.undp.org/content/dam/undp/library/HIV-AIDS/NCDs/Legislators%20English.pdf

3 Samira Humaira Habib and Soma Saha, 'Burden of Non-Communicable Disease: Global Overview', *Diabetes and Metabolic Syndrome: Clinical Research and Reviews*, 4.1 (2010), 41–47, https://doi.org/10.1016/j.dsx.2008.04.005

4 World Health Organization, 'United Nations High-Level Meeting on Non-communicable Disease Prevention and Control', 2011, https://www.who.int/nmh/events/un_ncd_summit2011/en/; World Health Organization, 'High-Level Meeting of the UN General Assembly to Undertake the Comprehensive Review and Assessment of the 2011 Political Declaration on NCDs', 2014, https://www.who.int/nmh/events/2014/high-level-unga/en/; World Health Organization, 'Third

 https://doi.org/10.11647/OBP.0195.02

take on individual and collective health outcomes and affirmed that preventing and controlling NCDs is essential to national, regional and global development. These political actions have been supported and reinforced by substantive technical guidance. For example, following the UN's Political Declaration on NCDs in 2011, WHO developed a global monitoring framework[5] and identified sixteen Best Buy interventions as part of the 2013 Global Action Plan for Prevention and Control of NCDs.[6] UN Member States now also receive support to collect and analyze surveillance data on NCDs.[7]

However, the continued rise of NCDs shows that increased political attention and knowledge of prevention strategies has yet to translate into effective policy implementation at national and local levels. For example, the cost-effectiveness of prevention has been demonstrated broadly, including in the WHO 2018 'Saving lives, spending less' report.[8] The United Nations Development Programme (UNDP), in collaboration with WHO, has also developed briefs on how multiple sectors can engage in the prevention of NCDs.[9] Yet, NCDs receive less than 2% of all health funding globally,[10] and less than 1% in LMICs.[11] Additionally, as we explore in this chapter and has been shown in the Caribbean region,[12] NCD funding

---

United Nations High-Level Meeting on NCDs', 2018, https://www.who.int/ncds/governance/third-un-meeting/en/

5 World Health Organization, *NCD Global Monitoring Framework*, 2017, https://www.who.int/nmh/global_monitoring_framework/en/

6 World Health Organization, *Tackling NCDs: Best Buys*, 2017, http://apps.who.int/iris/bitstream/handle/10665/259232/WHO-NMH-NVI-17.9-eng.pdf?sequence=1

7 World Health Organization, *STEPwise Approach to Surveillance (STEPS)*, 2019, https://www.who.int/ncds/surveillance/steps/en/

8 World Health Organization, *Saving Lives, Spending Less: A Strategic Response to Non-communicable Diseases, 2018,* https://apps.who.int/iris/bitstream/handle/10665/272534/WHO-NMH-NVI-18.8-eng.pdf?ua=1

9 United Nations Development Programme, *What Government Ministries Need to Know about Non-Communicable Diseases*, 2019, https://www.undp.org/content/undp/en/home/librarypage/hiv-aids/what-government-ministries-need-to-know-about-non-communicable-diseases.html

10 World Health Organization, *Non-communicable Diseases and Their Risk Factors*, 2019, https://www.who.int/ncds/management/ncds-strategic-response/en/

11 World Health Organization, *Saving Lives, Spending Less: A Strategic Response to Non-communicable Diseases.*

12 W. Andy Knight and Dinah Hippolyte, *Keeping NCDs as a Political Priority in the Caribbean: A Political Economy Analysis of Non-Communicable Disease Policy-Making,* 2005, https://www.paho.org/hq/index.php?option=com_docman&view=download&category_slug=forum-key-stakeholders-on-ncd-advancing-ncd-agenda-caribbean-8-9-june-2015-7994&alias=36065-keeping-ncds-as-a-political-priority-caribbean-andy-knight-065&Itemid=270&lang=en

has been concentrated on ensuring political commitment, as opposed to implementation activities. In part, this gap reflects the challenge of the many contextual factors that affect NCDs. Universally applicable solutions for NCDs are in short supply because these diseases and their related risk factors are strongly influenced by cultures, habits, lifestyles and other circumstances, which have an impact on the distribution of NCDs observed at local level. Implementing global recommendations also requires investment in data capture and management, governance structures, political buy-in and other capacities that may not be present in many settings. These contextual challenges impede efforts to advance NCD policy and action at national levels. Understanding the constellation of activities required to address NCDs, and then adapting them appropriately to address local circumstances, requires deft political and technical negotiation as well as action.

In this chapter, we identify reasons why global policy recommendations to address NCDs have not translated easily into effective programs and action. We focus our research on the experiences of national NCD managers and their reflections on local capacity and challenges. NCD managers are typically located in a Ministry of Health and responsible for an NCD unit, with a mandate focused on NCDs. We reasoned that their position within ministries of health would give them insights into the institutional arrangements, interests and ideas involved in advancing or challenging NCD action. The chapter begins by presenting our methods, followed by an explanation of NCD units and the NCD manager position. We used the 'Three-I's' framework (institutions, ideas and interests), to structure our findings and concluded with recommendations for NCD program managers and others for advancing progress against NCDs.

2.2 Methods for Interviews and Analysis

We gathered data by conducting semi-structured interviews with national NCD managers, representatives from WHO and civil society organizations and urban-level implementers. The interview guide (available in the Online Appendix 2)[13] was organized around three themes: priority-setting, work patterns and context. First, we asked about prioritization and allocation of resources for NCDs

13 Available at https://hdl.handle.net/20.500.12434/09617d51

(including staffing, money and political attention). Second, we elicited descriptions of how NCD managers and others in related positions work, including how they organized their own work and engaged other stakeholders within the Ministry of Health and other ministries, as well as patient groups and civil society groups. Third, we asked about successes achieved and challenges faced in order to gather information about factors and conditions that had influenced their outcomes. Throughout, we sought to understand how and why actions by NCD managers and units were (or were not) translated into NCD prevention and control.

Informants were identified by several means. We consulted NCD experts at the Health Intervention and Technology Assessment Program (HITAP) of the Ministry of Public Health of Thailand. In connection with Chapter 4, HITAP had solicited case studies from NCD managers on Best Buys, Wasted Buys and Contestable Buys; we issued interview invitations to the authors of approximately one-quarter of the cases. We also networked with contacts at the Harvard T. H. Chan School of Public Health and WHO to reach other possible interviewees.

In total, seventeen NCD experts agreed to an interview. We began each interview with an explanation of the project and pledged not to report personally identifying information without obtaining express permission. Of the interviewees, five were women and twelve were men. Eight were from the Asia/Pacific region (Bangladesh, Bhutan, China, Myanmar, Philippines (x2), Sri Lanka and Thailand); three from the Americas (Ecuador, Mexico and the Pan-American Health Organization regional office); three from Europe (Finland, Georgia and the WHO European Regional Office); and three from Africa (Ethiopia, Guinea and Kenya). Among our respondents were one NCD program implementer (Asia/Pacific region) and two who commented on regional considerations. A large majority (fourteen) of the interviewees were physicians. The others had backgrounds in health-related academia, consulting, or research positions. Fourteen interviews were carried out in English and three in Spanish. The interviews lasted for approximately twenty to forty minutes and were conducted via the internet and telephone.

To structure our findings, we chose the 3-I's framework: Institutions, Interests and Ideas. This analytical framework from the field of political science uses the 3-I's to describe processes involved in public policy development[14]. According to the framework, 'Institutions' represent the structures and norms that influence political behavior. These include issues of governance, mandates, mechanisms of accountability and hierarchical structures. We use the 'Institutions' category to describe and analyze the NCD unit structure, its position within national ministries of health and its relationships with other ministries and relevant stakeholders. The 'Interests' component represents stakeholders affected by the policies in question and their respective agendas. Taking account of interests also requires sensitivity to power dynamics among and between stakeholders, and the successes and failures the stakeholders may experience. For the purposes of this chapter, we interpret interests as incorporating the various sectors involved in NCD action, including those that are not formal health services, with their own particular influences and preoccupations. 'Ideas', lastly, represents evidence, knowledge and the values of all policy makers, stakeholders and the public. 'Ideas' also includes ways to represent NCD policies and global recommendations for the advancement of NCDs at national level.

2.3 Institutions: NCD Managers, NCD Units and Ministries of Health

We were told that NCD units (and also NCD Divisions or NCD Programs) are recent bodies in national ministries of health.[15] Over 50%

14 National Collaborating Centre for Health Public Policy, *Understanding Policy Developments and Choices Through the '3-i' Framework: Interests, Ideas, and Institutions*, 2014, http://www.ncchpp.ca/docs/2014_procpp_3iframework_en.pdf; N. Bashir and W. Ungar, *The 3-I Framework: A Framework for Developing Policies Regarding Pharmacogenomics (PGx) Testing in Canada. Genome.*, 2015, https://tspace.library.utoronto.ca/bitstream/1807/70678/1/gen-2015-0100.pdf

15 Interview 1, 'Consultant, Ministry of Health, Asia-Pacific Region,' Skype interview, 29 November 2018; Interview 2, 'Advisor, Ministry of Health, European Region,' WhatsApp interview, 20 December 2018; Interview 3, 'NCD Manager, Ministry of Health, African Region,' WhatsApp interview, 18 December 2018; Interview 4, 'NCDs Program Advisor, Ministry of Health, African Region,' Skype interview, 18 December 2018; Interview 5, 'NCD Program Manager, Ministry of Health, African Region,' WhatsApp interview, 18 December 2018; Interview 6, 'Former Director of Technical Support Body, Ministry of Health, Asia-Pacific Region,' Skype interview, 24 January 2019; Interview 7, 'Program Officer, Ministry of Health, Asia-Pacific,' Skype interview, 8 March 2019; Interview 8, 'Advisor for NCDs, Regional Organization,' Skype interview, 12 March 2019; Interview 9, 'Senior Official, Ministry of Health, Americas Region,' Skype interview, 18 February 2019; Interview 10, 'Senior Official, Ministry of Health, Americas Region,' Skype

of the NCD units and programs whose managers and representatives we interviewed had been established in the early 2010s,[16] and all informants reported that attention to NCDs had increased in the past five to ten years in their countries. They cited various reasons for this, beginning with the rising NCD burdens brought on by aging populations and increased exposure to risk factors, noting that 'risk factors are easier to identify and target [with vertical mechanisms]'.[17] Tools, guidelines and frameworks produced over this period such as the Package of Essential NCD interventions (WHO PEN)[18] and the STEPswise approach to surveillance (STEPs) surveys[19] by WHO were also referenced as influential in increasing the attention paid to NCDs. On average, NCD managers had worked in their positions for close to nine years, with many having been appointed when the unit was established or shortly thereafter. The average number of employees in the NCD units or related programs in our sample was seventeen, with a range of nine to fifty (excluding front-line providers and implementers). All respondents reported having between one and three people working on NCDs at a managerial level. We were not able to learn exactly how this compares with the number of staff dedicated to communicable diseases, although our interviewees indicated that it was higher than for NCDs.

Interviewees reported that ministries of health were generally organized in two broad divisions: one was responsible for public health and health promotion, and the other had a mandate for service delivery

interview, 12 April 2019; Interview 11, 'Officer, Multilateral Organization, Asia-Pacific Region,' in-person interview, 1 February 2019; Interview 12, 'Former Officer, Multilateral Organization, Asia-Pacific Region,' in-person interview, 1 February 2019; Interview 13, 'NCD Department Head, Ministry of Health, European Region,' Skype interview, 12 April 2019; Interview 14, 'Country Representative, Multilateral Organization, Asia-Pacific Region,' Skype interview, 15 March 2019; Interview 15, 'NCD Division Director, Regional Organization,' Skype interview, 15 March 2019; Interview 16, 'NCD Program Coordinator, City-Level, Ministry of Health, Asia-Pacific Region,' Skype interview, 28 March 2019; Interview 17, 'Senior Official, Ministry of Health, Asia-Pacific Region,' Facebook Messenger interview, 8 May 2019.

16 Interview 1; Interview 3; Interview 4; Interview 5; Interview 7; Interview 8; Interview 9; Interview 10; Interview 15.

17 Interview 15.

18 World Health Organization, *Tools for Implementing WHO PEN (Package of Essential Non-communicable Disease Interventions)*, 2019, https://www.who.int/ncds/management/pen_tools/en/

19 World Health Organization, *STEPwise Approach to Surveillance (STEPS).*

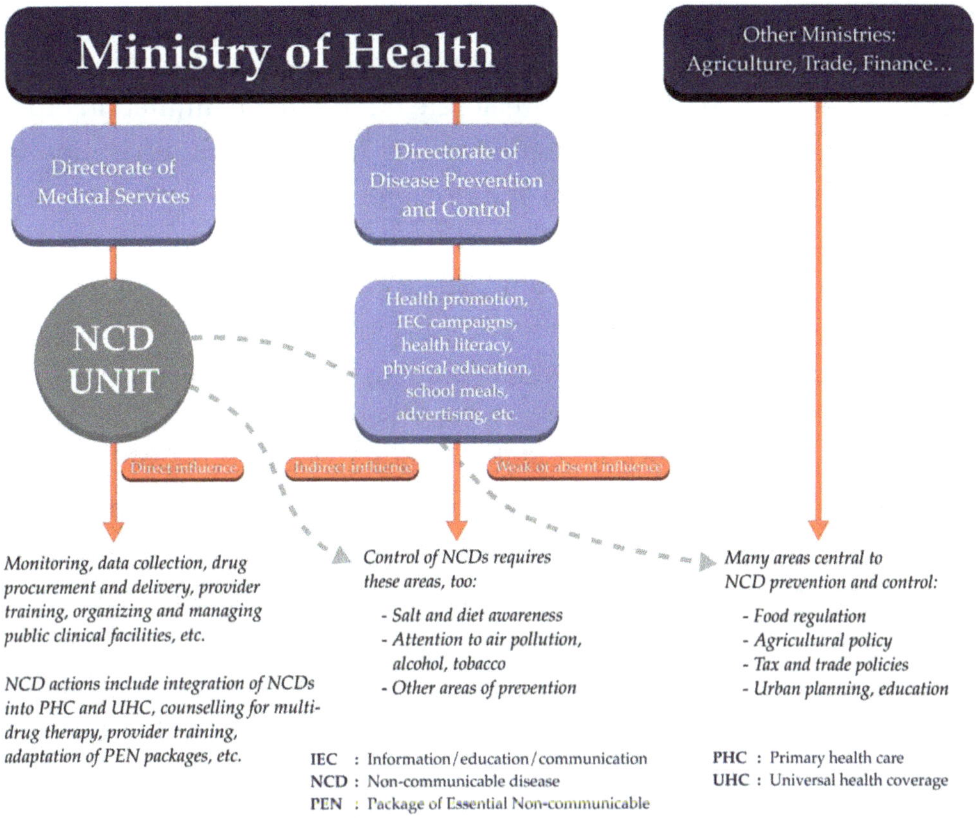

Fig. 2.1 Ministry of Health Organization and consequences for NCD Units.

and disease control. In over 40% of our cases, the NCD units (inclusive of two NCD divisions, one national and one regional)[20] were located in the service delivery and disease control division or directorates. In these cases, respondents explicitly noted that the NCD units did not oversee the management of risk factors, such as tobacco smoking, alcohol use and dietary improvement; these were instead addressed either in the Ministry's health promotion or public health directorates, or in separate units. Two countries[21] in our sample had no specific NCD units or program, three had NCD units or programs that sat in the disease prevention and control directorates,[22] two sat in public health or prevention and promotion directorates[23] and one division sat under

20 Interview 3; Interview 5; Interview 6; Interview 8; Interview 11; Interview 12; Interview 14.

21 Interview 2; Interview 10.

22 Interview 4; Interview 9; Interview 16; Interview 17.

23 Interview 7; Interview 13.

direct regional administration.[24] As shown in Figure 2.1, the placement of the NCD unit inside a larger directorate has consequences for its influence — strong within the directorate but relatively limited in other directorates, which was also mentioned by interviewees in relation to authority over NCD risk factors and preventive action.

We were told that the mandates of the NCD units were reflected in national NCD policies and action plans. These task NCD units with responsibility for diseases that vary according to the country that was reporting. Some NCDs were common to all countries, such as cardiovascular diseases, diabetes, hypertension and cancers. Others, for example, rheumatic disease,[25] sickle cell disease[26] and eye health,[27] were mentioned in only one or two countries. Other cited NCDs addressed by the NCD units and national plans included chronic kidney disease,[28] mental health,[29] neurological diseases,[30] asthma,[31] genetic diseases[32] and renal diseases.[33] Interviewees also mentioned NCD policies encompassing elderly care,[34] injury prevention,[35] urgent care,[36] palliative care[37] and drug and substance abuse.[38] Commenting on the breadth of NCDs covered, one manager suggested that 'even the concept of "NCDs" is a problem [...] it is not easy to understand [...] it seems too large'.[39] In turn, because of this large scope 'the challenges [NCD managers] have [are] on coordination'.[40] Figure 2.2 below summarizes the frequency with which particular NCDs were mentioned as a proportion of interviews in which they were cited.

---

24 Interview 15.
25 Interview 4.
26 Interview 5.
27 Interview 4; Interview 17.
28 Interview 1; Interview 4; Interview 7; Interview 8.
29 Interview 2; Interview 4; Interview 5; Interview 6; Interview 8; Interview 12; Interview 13; Interview 14; Interview 15; Interview 16; Interview 17.
30 Interview 4; Interview 14.
31 Interview 4; Interview 9; Interview 16.
32 Interview 15.
33 Interview 1; Interview 16.
34 Interview 3; Interview 16.
35 Interview 8; Interview 13; Interview 14; Interview 15; Interview 16.
36 Interview 14; Interview 15.
37 Interview 7.
38 Interview 17.
39 Interview 5.
40 Interview 5.

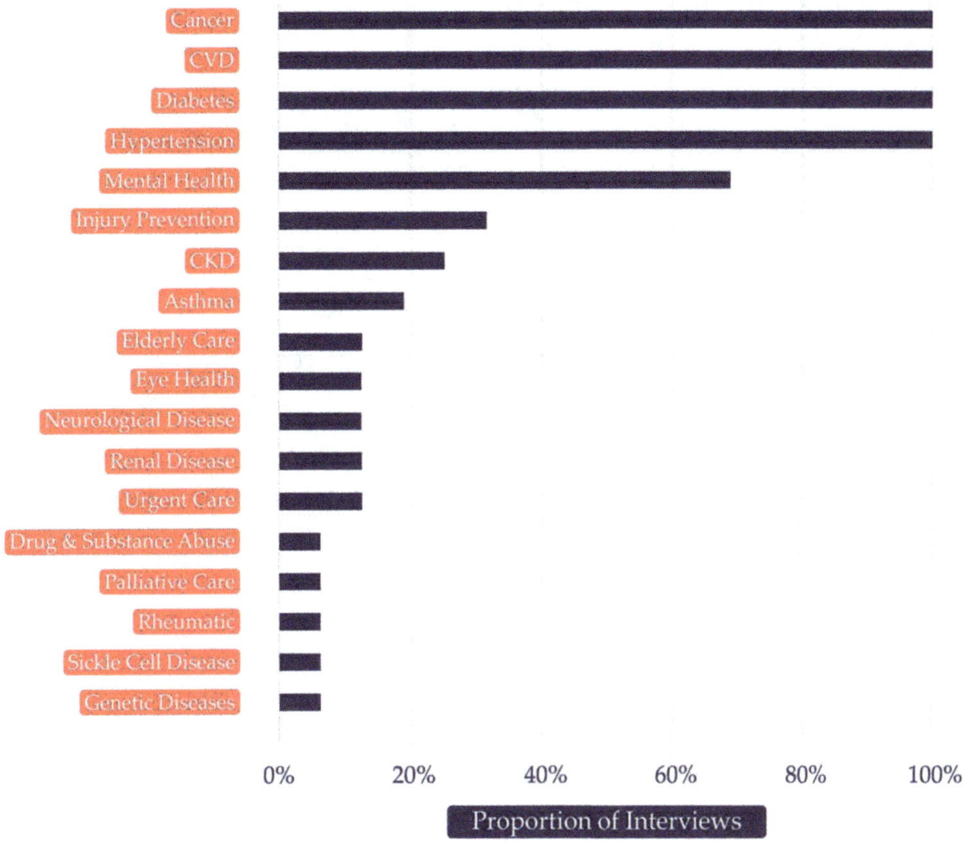

Fig. 2.2 NCDs ranked by proportion of interviews in which they were mentioned.

Nearly 40% of respondents reported that cancers were dealt with differently from other NCDs.[41] Reasons included the high funding demands for cancer and the need for stronger health system capacity to address cancer incidence. Respondents also noted that cancer management requires control over risk factors, such as air pollution, that cannot be addressed by NCD units or ministries of health alone, requiring the engagement and support of other ministries and stakeholders — the Ministry of Environment and polluting industries were cited, among others.

The NCD units included in our sample were engaged in a broad set of activities, ranging from raising awareness about NCDs to designing NCD policies and programs. In nearly 90% of the country cases in our sample, NCD units were responsible for technical coordination, capacity

41 Interview 3; Interview 7; Interview 9; Interview 10; Interview 14; Interview 17.

building and training of health personnel, advocacy and awareness-raising. Most respondents also described undertaking activities such as the creation of tools and recommendations for training front-line providers in provincial centers and integrating NCD screening into health services. Data collection and monitoring, through STEPS surveys, Burden of Disease Studies[42] and Disease Control Priorities Project[43] (DCP3), were also cited as key responsibilities of nearly all NCD units in our sample. However, no national or regional NCD units were directly involved in implementation efforts, as these were responsibilities carried out by other stakeholders, including other ministries, local health officers and civil society organizations.[44] Additionally, in most of the sampled countries, legislative processes precede the implementation of NCD efforts operationally and in priority.

2.4 Interests: Stakeholders and Power

The complex multiple causal pathways of NCDs are influenced by many sectors beyond health care,[45] including trade, agriculture and education, making multisectoral coordination especially important. All of our respondents recognized that, for NCD prevention in particular, approaches often fall outside the scope of ministries of health, with one interviewee reflecting that tobacco and alcohol industries 'are tackled with the muscle of other institutions.'[46] All respondents similarly emphasized the importance of multisectoral engagement and political buy-in for implementation efforts. Examples of stakeholders with whom NCD managers and units work, particularly for the implementation of NCD policy, include other national ministries, the private sector and

42 Global Burden of Disease Collaborative Network, *Global Burden of Disease Study 2017* (Seattle, United States: Institute for Health Metrics and Evaluation (IHME), 2019), http://ghdx.healthdata.org/gbd-results-tool

43 Disease Control Priorities: Economic evaluation for health, *DCP3*, 2019, http://dcp-3.org/

44 Interview 1; Interview 2; Interview 3; Interview 4; Interview 5; Interview 6; Interview 7; Interview 8; Interview 9; Interview 10; Interview 11; Interview 12; Interview 13; Interview 14; Interview 15; Interview 17.

45 World Health Organization; Regional Office for the Eastern Mediterranean, *Non-communicable Diseases,* 2019, http://www.emro.who.int/noncommunicable-diseases/publications/questions-and-answers-on-the-multisectoral-action-plan-to-prevent-and-control-noncommunicable-diseases-in-the-region.html

46 Interview 3.

civil society. Respondents also acknowledged receiving funding and technical support from international organizations such as WHO, NCD Alliance, Partners in Health, PATH (the global health nonprofit), the United States Agency for International Development (USAID), Japan International Cooperation Agency (JICA) and the World Bank. WHO was cited by all respondents as an active contributor to the advancement of NCDs in national policy agendas and as helping to raise awareness of NCD burdens. More than one-third of interviewees reported that their countries had adopted the WHO PEN[47] and had begun at least partial implementation. The WHO's recommendations on restrictions on tobacco and alcohol through the Framework Convention on Tobacco Control (FCTC)[48] and the Global Strategy to Reduce the Harmful Use of Alcohol[49] had also been considered, with nearly 60% of the countries in the sample having enacted legislation in at least one of these areas[50] and the remaining countries working to do so.

NCD managers and units engaged with vested stakeholders in several different ways across our sample countries, and no two countries reported having the same multi-stakeholder engagement model. Some respondents used roundtable discussions, focus groups and research collaborations. Nearly one-quarter of the respondents reported that NCD action in their countries was overseen by multisectoral committees in which authority and decision-making was rotated and shared among members;[51] this structure was specifically cited for the oversight of key risk factors such as unhealthy diets and tobacco use. Two interviewees reported participating in parliamentary procedures including voting and proposing policy motions, with the Ministry of Health holding ultimate authority.[52] Other examples of multi-stakeholder collaborations included working with the Road Safety Ministry to introduce alcohol

47 Interview 5; Interview 7; Interview 11; Interview 12; Interview 16; Interview 17; World Health Organization, *Tools for Implementing WHO PEN (Package of Essential Non-communicable Disease Interventions)*.

48 World Health Organization, *Framework Convention on Tobacco Control*, 2003, https://apps.who.int/iris/bitstream/handle/10665/42811/9241591013.pdf?sequence=1

49 World Health Organization, *Global Strategy to Reduce the Harmful Use of Alcohol. World Health Organization*, 2010, https://apps.who.int/iris/handle/10665/44395

50 Interview 1; Interview 2; Interview 4; Interview 6; Interview 11; Interview 13; Interview 14; Interview 15; Interview 16, Interview 17.

51 Interview 2; Interview 6; Interview 10; Interview 13.

52 Interview 2; Interview 13.

breathalyzers,[53] the introduction of food labeling requirements with the Ministry of Agriculture,[54] the promotion of physical activity and healthier diets with and in schools,[55] and engaging with the media for mass health promotion campaigns.[56]

In terms of institutional arrangements for action on NCDs, our respondents reported that decision-making authority usually sat with Ministers of Health or political leaders, stipulating that their role and units '[have] little authority',[57] 'are weak'[58] and 'are not in [a] strong position'.[59] Almost all of our interviewees suggested that political leaders were in charge of both funding allocation and priority-setting in national agendas; in these cases, NCDs were competing with other health priorities, and the Ministry of Health was competing with other ministries for attention and resources. As a result, NCD managers reported resorting to knowledge-building and awareness-raising about NCDs, specifically targeted at politicians and Ministers of Health. Ultimately, NCD managers reported that the NCD units alone hold little authority or oversight over setting priorities or making decisions at a national level.

While our respondents recognized the importance of multi-stakeholder engagement, it was cited as a challenge by nearly half of them. About 30% (five out of seventeen respondents) mentioned a lack of coordination of multi-stakeholder meetings and strategies,[60] and three managers suggested that NCD action appears daunting and/or confusing to non-experts.[61] Some respondents suggested that further guidance and models could help improve multi-stakeholder engagement.

2.5 Ideas: Evidence, Knowledge and Values

How countries engage in NCD action arguably reflects how NCDs are perceived in that setting. Some NCD managers noted that 'ten

53 Interview 7.
54 Interview 7; Interview 10; Interview 17.
55 Interview 1; Interview 2; Interview 5; Interview 9.
56 Interview 1; Interview 6; Interview 10; Interview 13.
57 Interview 6.
58 Interview 5.
59 Ibid.
60 Interview 1; Interview 4; Interview 5; Interview 14; Interview 17.
61 Interview 3; Interview 5; Interview 15.

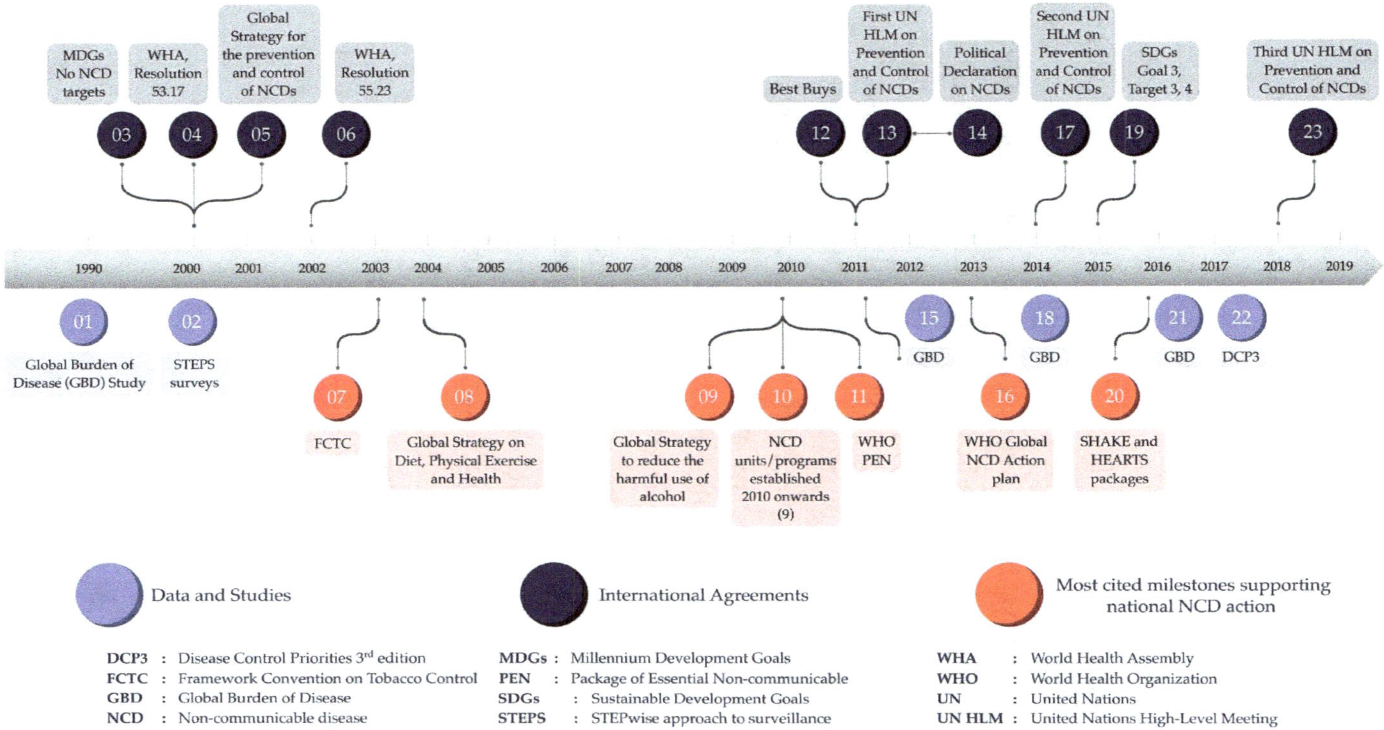

Fig. 2.3 Timeline of milestones in NCD action from 1990–2019.

years ago, we [at the national level] did not have any official interest in NCDs,'[62] and that attention to risk factors preceded attention to the burden of NCDs, as evidenced by historical efforts. To illustrate the changes in attention to NCDs over the last few decades, we developed a timeline (Fig. 2.3) which highlights international agreements, data and monitoring methods and key milestones that were cited as particularly important by interviewees in achieving national NCD action from legislation to implementation.

The decade of 2000–2010 was 'marked by a rebellion against the neglect of the NCDs in the MDGs',[63] and our interviewees held a mixed assessment of how NCDs were currently being prioritized in their countries. Five respondents judged that NCDs were considered a low priority[64] with one reporting that 'NCDs don't get the attention they deserve considering [the] deaths and morbidity they cause'.[65] In contrast, six believed that their countries gave them high priority.[66] Across our sample, prioritization among NCDs also varied; cardiovascular disease was cited as the top priority NCD by six interviewees.[67] Within the NCD agenda, mental health,[68] injury prevention,[69] palliative care[70] and kidney issues[71] were reportedly gaining increasing attention. Some respondents underscored the poor attention given to chronic respiratory diseases.[72] In dealing with NCDs at a broader level, seven respondents reported that service provision was, or should be, a higher priority than prevention.[73] Service provision examples mentioned included coverage at district level, capacity building and training of service providers, drug procurement, early detection and integration of NCD services with primary care and universal health coverage and, as already reported,

62 Interview 5.
63 Interview 15.
64 Interview 3; Interview 4; Interview 5; Interview 13; Interview 16.
65 Interview 3.
66 Interview 1; Interview 2; Interview 7; Interview 9; Interview 10; Interview 17.
67 Interview 4; Interview 8; Interview 12; Interview 13; Interview 14; Interview 15.
68 Interview 2; Interview 4; Interview 6; Interview 8; Interview 12; Interview 13; Interview 14; Interview 15; Interview 16; Interview 17.
69 Interview 8; Interview 13; Interview 14; Interview 15; Interview 16.
70 Interview 7.
71 Interview 1; Interview 4; Interview 6; Interview 7; Interview 8.
72 Interview 9; Interview 14; Interview 15.
73 Interview 1; Interview 3; Interview 5; Interview 6; Interview 13; Interview 16; Interview 17.

service provision received larger budget allocations than prevention in nearly half the units in our sample.

Regarding the prioritization of risk factors, all interviewees highlighted the importance of interventions to promote healthy diets and exercise. Efforts to promote diet and exercise included advertising,[74] taxation,[75] and educational campaigns.[76] One interviewee described an effort to establish outdoor gyms.[77] Actions against tobacco and/or alcohol use were cited in nearly 65% of interviews,[78] typically in relation to legislation and surveillance. Other risk factors mentioned were air pollution,[79] chewing tobacco[80] and salt consumption.[81] Generally, action for salt reduction lags behind the more common measures for addressing alcohol and tobacco use.

Interviewees described the importance of perception of NCDs in relation to the implementation and uptake of interventions. Factors affecting public perception cited by managers included the influence of politicians in two decision-making settings,[82] social networks in five,[83] and media in four.[84] These factors reportedly influenced attitudes towards screening, healthier diets and health literacy.

In nearly 60% of our interviews, concerns were expressed that the implementation of NCD action lacked buy-in from politicians and stakeholders,[85] with some respondents suggesting that NCDs were 'not a real priority, only a priority on paper'.[86] For example, seven interviewees mentioned problems in enforcing legislation.[87] Although

74 Interview 1; Interview 3; Interview 5; Interview 13; Interview 16; Interview 17.

75 Interview 2; Interview 6; Interview 9; Interview 10; Interview 11; Interview 17.

76 Interview 1; Interview 2; Interview 4; Interview 5; Interview 10.

77 Interview 7.

78 Interview 1; Interview 2; Interview 4; Interview 6; Interview 8; Interview 10; Interview 13; Interview 14; Interview 15; Interview 16; Interview 17.

79 Interview 2; Interview 4; Interview 9; Interview 13; Interview 14.

80 Interview 4; Interview 11.

81 Interview 4; Interview 6; Interview 7; Interview 8; Interview 11; Interview 13; Interview 14; Interview 16.

82 Interview 3; Interview 4.

83 Interview 1; Interview 2; Interview 5; Interview 7; Interview 13.

84 Interview 1; Interview 6; Interview 10; Interview 13.

85 Interview 2; Interview 3; Interview 4; Interview 5; Interview 6; Interview 9; Interview 14; Interview 15; Interview 16; Interview 17.

86 Interview 6.

87 Interview 3; Interview 4; Interview 5; Interview 6; Interview 12; Interview 15; Interview 17.

all countries in our sample had cited the adoption of legislation for controlling tobacco and most other risk factors, four respondents[88] noted that there had been limited follow-through, little or no enforcement and few dedicated human or financial resources. Other challenges that were mentioned as impeding action on NCDs included the inability to control the inflow and outflow of potentially harmful substances,[89] and weak advocacy efforts.[90] Six interviewees cited cultural and behavioral inertia as a challenge.[91] This inertia was related in some cases to links between religious practices and carbohydrate consumption,[92] perceptions of junk-food consumption as a sign of modernization and prosperity,[93] or reliance on neighbors and family members for health information.[94] It was also suggested that the delegation of responsibilities outside the NCD unit and Ministry of Health created challenges.

Reflections from respondents were mixed in terms of effective and successful implementation of Best Buys. This finding is relevant because Best Buy recommendations are predominantly focused on risk factor action, which underscores the focus on service delivery by NCD units and the challenges in relation to multisectoral coordination that have already been highlighted. While all respondents reported that the recommended alcohol and tobacco legislation was in place, only five respondents[95] mentioned implementation of the salt consumption recommendation and a mere two[96] mentioned vaccination against human papillomavirus. In one country, drug therapy and counselling services were reported to be available for individuals with diabetes, hypertension, or a history of heart attack or stroke.[97] Smoke-free public spaces were cited by four interviewees,[98] health information and warnings about tobacco by five,[99] and bans on alcohol advertising and

88 Interview 3; Interview 4; Interview 5; Interview 6.
89 Interview 2.
90 Interview 5; Interview 13.
91 Interview 1; Interview 4; Interview 5; Interview 9; Interview 13; Interview 14.
92 Interview 1.
93 Interview 5.
94 Interview 13.
95 Interview 4; Interview 6; Interview 7; Interview 11; Interview 17.
96 Interview 13; Interview 16.
97 Interview 16; Interview 17.
98 Interview 6; Interview 10; Interview 16; Interview 17.
99 Interview 6; Interview 10; Interview 12; Interview 16; Interview 17.

restricted access to retail alcohol by two.[100] Trans fats were cited by three respondents,[101] but with no implementation. Mass-media campaigns relating to diet and physical activity were reported by six interviewees.[102] Some suggested that the implementation of Best Buys would benefit from detailed recommendations for implementation at the local level.[103] Five respondents also suggested that the Best Buys need to be more sensitive to context.[104] Noting that 'Best Buys are useful to define national priorities, but are not automatic',[105] some interviewees felt that Best Buys are too 'broad'[106] and should consider context-specific capacity and needs, especially as 'what works in one country is not transferable'.[107] Respondents also cited other policies as Best Buys, such as the PEN[108] and HEARTS[109] (technical package for cardiovascular disease management in primary health care) packages, as well as school meals, though these are not officially designated as Best Buys by the WHO.[110]

2.6 Discussion

Why have global recommendations and guidance on how to advance action on NCDs not been easily translated into improvements in local health outcomes? Understanding the reasons behind the generally reported difficulties involves examining institutional arrangements of NCD units within ministries, the varied interests of relevant stakeholders and the diverse ideas shaping perceptions of NCDs. Overall, our findings highlight many positive improvements in the recognition of NCDs in national agendas. The informants attributed this development to the combination of emphasis placed on NCDs by global bodies and

100 Interview 6; Interview 13.
101 Interview 7; Interview 9; Interview 16.
102 Interview 1; Interview 5; Interview 6; Interview 10; Interview 13; Interview 16.
103 Interview 2; Interview 4; Interview 9; Interview 14; Interview 15.
104 Ibid.
105 Interview 9.
106 Ibid.
107 Interview 2.
108 World Health Organization, *Tools for Implementing WHO PEN (Package of Essential Non-communicable Disease Interventions).*
109 World Health Organization, *Hearts: Technical Package for Cardiovascular Disease Management in Primary Health Care, 2016,* https://apps.who.int/iris/bitstream/handle/10665/252661/9789241511377-eng.pdf?sequence=1
110 Interview 7; Interview 10; Interview 16; Interview 17.

advocates, changes in population profiles and growing epidemiological evidence of the burden of NCDs. National developments, such as the establishment of NCD units, the adoption of frameworks and policies based on internationally determined good practices, and expanding efforts to collect data on NCDs, were increasingly evident. Furthermore, the types of NCD policies adopted by national governments were largely guided by global-level leadership from WHO. We see these developments as positive examples of global recommendations and stakeholders influencing local agendas and action on NCDs. However, according to NCD managers, many challenges remain, which expose the need for increasing the adaptability of global recommendations to local levels.

The institutional arrangements of NCD units, like service provision divisions of ministries of health, may not be adequate for the adaptation and adoption of global recommendations. For example, many of these recommendations and guidelines, including Best Buy recommendations, address both service delivery and prevention, some aspects of which are outside the mandate of service providers. Moreover, NCDs tend not to have single-cause origins or etiologies and thus cannot be interrupted directly, as is possible with many infectious diseases.[111] In some instances, the distinction between prevention and service delivery is not clear, as when addressing diabetes incidence and prevalence by promoting exercise,[112] or cases in which chemotherapy is used preventively for certain cancers.[113] Some institutional arrangements further limit how global recommendations can support the coordination of prevention efforts. Locating NCD units in service provision strengthens the service delivery components of NCD action. While useful, this structure can, however, separate NCD managers from the overall scope of multisectoral preventive efforts in their own views and the views of other stakeholders.

---

111 Center for Disease Control, *Overview of Non-communicable Diseases and Related Risk Factors*, 2013, https://www.cdc.gov/globalhealth/healthprotection/fetp/training_modules/new-8/Overview-of-NCDs_PPT_QA-RevCom_09112013.pdf

112 Igor P. Briazgounov, 'The Role of Physical Activity in the Prevention and Treatment of Noncommunicable Diseases', *World Health Statistics Quarterly*, 41.3–4 (1988), 242–50.

113 Science Direct, *Adjuvant Chemotherapy*, 2017, https://www.sciencedirect.com/topics/medicine-and-dentistry/adjuvant-chemotherapy

The institutional mandates of NCD units often require engaging with a broad range of risk factors and activities. Global recommendations do not fully recognize the multitude of tasks that fall to NCD units. For example, the HEARTS[114] and SHAKE technical package for salt reduction[115] target individual diseases and risk factors; they do not include activities that address the overall mandates of NCD units. The heterogeneity (among countries) and diversity (within countries) of the challenges that contribute to NCDs make it difficult for global actors to promote consistently compelling messages and effective policies.

Grouping all NCDs in one unit within a ministry contrasts starkly with the prevailing practice for addressing infectious diseases. A ministry generally comprises many units, some responsible for a single disease (such as malaria or tuberculosis) and some presiding over a group of related diseases (such as sexually transmitted infections). The breadth of diseases designated for the NCD unit creates operational challenges. One of our informants mentioned that 'there's a lot of debate about what NCDs are',[116] which we interpret to underscore the difficulty of developing technical competence and strategic partnerships across a large portfolio of NCDs, which vary from country to country. Furthermore, it generates challenges in the ways in which NCDs are perceived by stakeholders, potentially exacerbating confusion and frustration in the time-frame required to see results. Political influence and buy-in to address the full range of NCDs is also especially difficult, given the complexities involved and the inherent competing priorities. A similar challenge arises from trying to address an array of diseases without duplicating efforts, which could be particularly difficult for NCDs located within disease-prevention-and-control directorates. Finally, the funding and staffing allocations for NCD units were generally low, especially when compared with communicable disease units.

The difficulties engendered by the institutional arrangements and mandates of NCD units are underscored by a lack of evidence on

114 World Health Organization, *Hearts: Technical Package for Cardiovascular Disease Management in Primary Health Care.*

115 World Health Organization, *The SHAKE Technical Package for Salt Reduction,* 2016, https://apps.who.int/iris/bitstream/handle/10665/250135/9789241511346-eng.pdf?sequence=1

116 Interview 14.

best practices for coordinating the interests of multiple stakeholders. Although we found it encouraging that all interviewees reported that NCD units work with various stakeholders on implementation, prevention and risk reduction, among other activities, the effectiveness of such engagements has not been well documented. One manager suggested that 'the NCD community [...] are not yet embracing health systems components'[117] and others expressed a need for frameworks or other guidance on how to engage stakeholders successfully for coordinated action. Existing efforts, including available tools[118] and documents,[119] have not yet been widely mainstreamed nor have they been especially relevant in national settings.

The diversity of stakeholders with whom NCD units sought to engage reflects the breadth of concerns and risk factors connected with NCDs. For a unit with just one, two, or three managerial positions, coordination across the full range of stakeholders for NCDs represents a monumental task. We identified a need for further research to develop guidance on organizing a bureaucracy for effective NCD action. This also highlights a gap in the existing global recommendations: identifying best practices for multi-stakeholder action to mainstream NCD action in recognition of the multiple demands NCD unit mandates have.

Respondents also stated that there was nearly always a strong focus on upstream action, such as legislative efforts or the development of national strategies. Relatively little focus was placed on downstream activities such as multisectoral coordination, with one interviewee noting that 'the solution is there, we just need to do it'.[120] An emphasis on upstream action could possibly be interpreted as a weak commitment to NCDs—after all, implementation is typically more resource-intensive than policy making. It could also indicate that the international guidelines and frameworks have focused too much on securing mandates rather than on supporting operational activities, which is underscored by one of our respondents reflecting that 'the time

117 Interview 14.

118 World Health Organization, *Toolkit for Developing, Implementing and Evaluation the National Multisectoral Action Plan (MAP) for NCD Prevention and Control*, 2019, http://apps.who.int/nmh/ncd-map-toolkit/index.html

119 World Health Organization, *Approaches to Establishing Country-Level Multisectoral Coordination Mechanisms for the Prevention and Control of Non-communicable Diseases'*, 2015.

120 Interview 1.

is now for implementation, not further standards and norm-setting'.[121] This is also reflected in our interviewees frequently discussing Best Buy recommendations in relation to legislative efforts with relatively low enforcement capacity. Poor enforcement of policies may result from a lack of focus on operational aspects or capacity, resulting in a lack of designated responsibility and corresponding accountability for implementation and enforcement. If the consequences of not enforcing a policy, including a lack of clarity about who is responsible, have not been clearly outlined, policies will not be effectively implemented. Ultimately, NCD managers might, in addition to their current roles, also be forced to take on responsibility for enforcement. Alternatively, they could develop strong liaisons with those delegated to implement in order to ensure buy-in and attention to NCD action. Incidentally, these interviewees reminded us that beyond the FCTC,[122] global action against commercial and environmental determinants of health has, as of yet, been modest.

Finally, the interviews revealed clearly that, while international advocacy and recommendations have successfully raised the level of attention given to NCDs in at least some countries, 'the challenge has now reduced itself to implementation, [requiring] a different set of skills'[123] to assist countries in contextualizing recommended approaches and adapting priorities to their specific needs. A major obstacle to such downstream actions was the limited knowledge and engagement that national political leaders demonstrated in relation to NCDs, as well as general ideas and perceptions of NCDs among government and population as a whole. To a large extent, global movements, rather than domestic advocacy, promoted NCDs within national policy agendas. Limited implementation of NCD policies at national level could also be interpreted as an indication of a disconnect between global and local perceptions of NCDs. NCD units and other advocates for NCD action need to build domestic support more systematically, including by educating national and local politicians. Additionally, the WHO should consider developing regionally contextualized recommendations that are easier for countries to use and adapt.

121 Interview 15.

122 World Health Organization, *Framework Convention on Tobacco Control.*

123 Interview 14.

2.7 Limitations

The research that informed this chapter had several limitations. First, despite extensive efforts over eight months to recruit interviewees, we received fewer positive responses than we wanted. A larger sample could have generated more, and more generalizable, conclusions. Second, although the interviewees represented a variety of countries and regions, the sample was skewed towards Asia, which made regional comparisons difficult. Third, the breadth and diversity of NCDs and settings encompassed in the interviews made it hard to investigate specific themes consistently. Fourth, the interview guide and the time allocated for interviews allowed for a high-level exploratory approach, as distinct from an exhaustive study of NCD efforts in the countries in our sample. Fifth, our interviews were not always conducted in the interviewees' first languages. This may have resulted in some confusion and limited the nuances of some responses. Finally, low-quality internet connections made some interviews especially difficult.

2.8 Conclusions and Recommendations

NCDs remain a key health-system challenge for virtually every country in the world.[124] Global NCD recommendations are rarely directly relevant and applicable to local settings. NCD units in national ministries of health face challenges in adopting and adapting global best practices to advance NCD action. These challenges arise from the mandates given to and institutional arrangements made for the units, the necessity of engaging with relevant stakeholders with diverse ideas and the difficulties inherent in prioritizing NCDs in relation to other national health and development plans. Nevertheless, encouraging developments are evident, particularly in the form of national legislation and other upstream actions. The WHO also has an important presence in local settings.

In our interviews with national NCD managers and similar actors, two needs were clearly revealed: first, support for stronger action

124 Ala Alawan, *The NCD Challenge: Progress in Responding to the Global NCD Challenge and the Way Forward*, 2017, https://www.who.int/nmh/events/2017/discussion-paper-for-the-ncd-who-meeting-final.pdf

downstream from the NCD unit; and second, improved frameworks for multi-stakeholder engagement and multisector coordination efforts. The implementation challenges reported by NCD managers revealed that additional leadership, resources and innovation were required. Meeting some of these needs lies beyond the remit and authority of either the NCD managers or ministries of health, outlining the ongoing role of global institutions and non-governmental organizations.

We propose three action points, based on our findings and analysis, that could support the translation of global NCD recommendations into better NCD outcomes at the local level:

- **Expand global support for engaging political leadership in NCD agendas.** NCD managers reported that the limited knowledge and engagement among senior political leaders was a major obstacle to prioritizing action on NCDs. We recommend developing advocacy guidance and materials for use by NCD managers. Technical experts, such as NCD managers, need simplified tools for educating and discussing key NCDs and related policies with potential advocacy partners (such as professional associations, patient groups and influential individuals who have personal experience with an NCD). Additionally, global institutions should use their access to senior politicians to create opportunities to conduct joint outreach and advocacy efforts. We recommend that global NCD advocates and experts collaborate with health ministers and NCD managers to identify one or more NCDs to emphasize and generate interest and action for relevant policies and programs.
- **Expand the managerial and institutional structures responsible for NCDs to reflect operational requirements and realities.** Most NCD units are not fully equipped or resourced to take on the complete range of NCDs and relevant activities. The placement of NCD units in either the public health or the service delivery division of the Ministry of Health represents a serious limitation. Even the attempt to narrow the programmatic approaches to pragmatic dimensions by identifying Best Buys still leaves NCD units with an extraordinarily wide range of activities to oversee. We

recommend that NCD units, ministries and global institutions consider expanding or creating parallel managerial structures aligned with the capacities needed to execute NCD programs. Alternatively, a simplification of the mandates of NCD units to target country-specific needs could facilitate managerial structures.

- **Generate effective guidance and support to stimulate multisectoral coordination, collaboration and action.** The NCD unit has little control or authority over the causes of and contributors to the vast majority of NCD risk factors. Although 'multisectoral action' has become a prominent buzzword of late, our interviews revealed that NCD managers neither had guidance on how to do it nor knew with precision what it was. However, NCD units are a natural focal point for discussing many multisectoral issues, such as tax policies for discouraging tobacco, alcohol and other harmful substances, and environmental protections to improve nutrition and food security. We recommend that NCD managers immediately begin pursuing informal relationships to foster such discussions, while global institutions develop specific, actionable and context-sensitive guidance for NCD managers on this topic.

3. Framework for Implementing Best Buys and Avoiding Wasted Buys

Yot Teerawattananon, Alia Luz, Manushi Sharma and Waranya Rattanavipapong

Best Buys and Wasted Buys are two sides of the same coin. If every healthcare system invested only in Best Buys, then Wasted Buys are automatically avoided. Therefore, if we understand the features of Best Buys, it is straightforward to understand the etiology of Wasted Buys. Best Buy policies are normally based on good intentions, rigorous evidence and efficient management and coordination; by contrast, Wasted Buy policies tend to be formulated with a weak rationale or self-interested motivation, absent or poor-quality evidence, inadequate management and weak coordination. Having a framework of step-by-step practical considerations to implementing Best Buys and avoiding Wasted Buys is consequently to have something of value. With this in mind, we propose the SEED Tool (Systematic thinking for Evidence-based and Efficient Decision-making) as shown in Figure 3.1.

The SEED Tool can be understood broadly in two parts: the inner circle and outer boxes. The inner circle is a set of fundamental questions that NCD policy managers and/or other decision-makers ought to ask themselves. NCD policy managers can increase the likelihood of implementing Best Buys and avoiding Wasted Buys if they systematically take account of each of these considerations. Each is numbered in a normative logical order. Interventions should ideally be assessed sequentially in the following order: sound theoretical basis (1), good quality evidence (2), transferability to the implementation setting (3), reasonable cost (4) and sufficient political investment (5). In practice,

 https://doi.org/10.11647/OBP.0195.03

however, NCD policy managers may order them differently, depending on their local and political contexts (e.g., starting from five, continuing on to three and then two, etc.). Provided that there are affirmative answers to each consideration, different orderings can still result in a Best Buy. To support this, the outer semi-circle has recommendations on how to incorporate and/or improve evidence support for each of the major considerations. It is important to note that this tool requires political commitment to using evidence for decision-making, which is separate from the political commitment to the intervention under scrutiny (see Consideration 5).

3.1 Consideration One

The first step questions the rationale or the theoretical background for the implementation of the intervention. Unlike curative interventions, where the effect can be observed early, NCD prevention interventions, as with most health-promotion and disease-prevention programs, have indirect effects on disease burdens. They aim to reduce health risks and therefore need a longer timeline to have any measurable impact on disease prevention. If programs do not use tested theories, they may not produce the desired improvements in health.[1] The strongest preventative programs have a clear conceptual basis that is built on good evidence. They guide the actual process of planning, implementation and evaluation. Understanding the purpose, history, constructs and context of the situation helps in selecting the most appropriate theory to guide the program. Preventive interventions also generally require commitment from individuals. For example, a mass media campaign to reduce obesity through healthy eating will be effective only if the target population understands and is responsive to the message. Governments can only promote the message but are unable to police healthy eating in the target population. As such, these policies require cultural understanding and should ideally be based on repeated proven experience in the field. This may involve a qualitative rather than a quantitative judgement but should nonetheless be one for which there is persuasive evidence.

1 Carl I. Fertman and Diane D. Allensworth, *Health Promotion Programs — From Theory to Practice*, 1st edn (San Francisco: Jossey-Bass, 2010), http://soh.iums.ac.ir/uploads/4.pdf

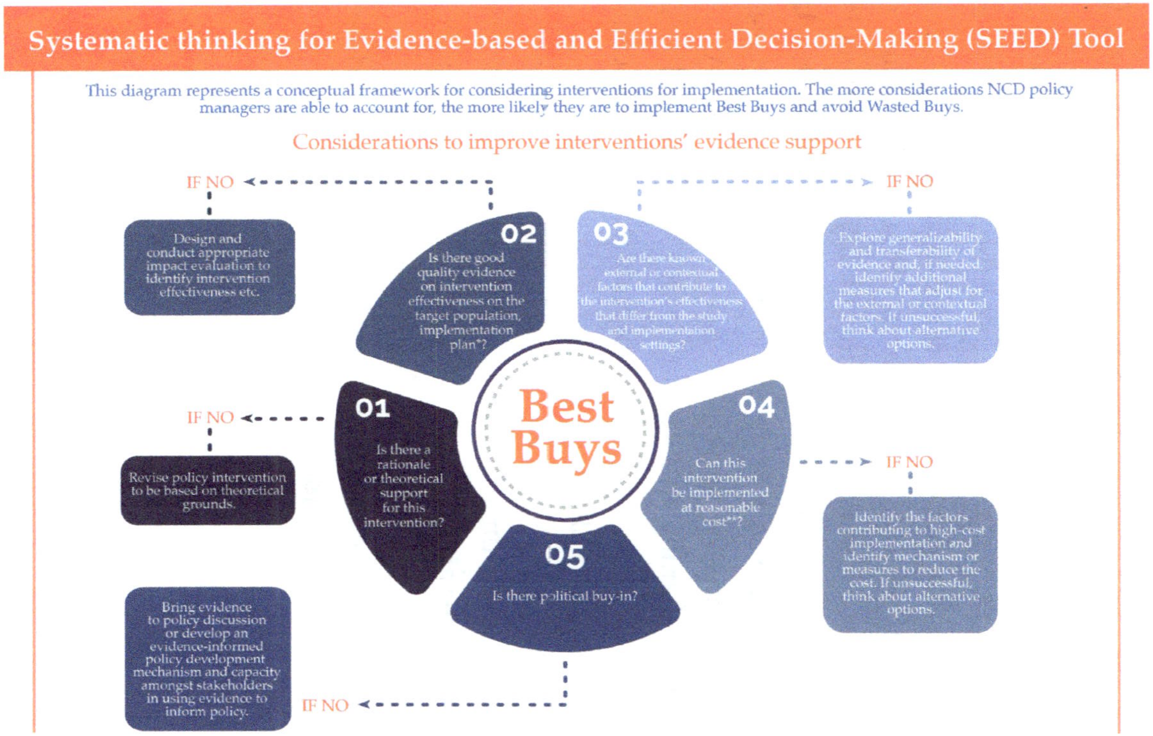

*Implementation = dosage, frequency, duration, coverage, etc.

**In comparison to the cost of implementing a similar program in other settings or compared to the cost parameters used in economic evaluation studies that led to a policy decision to adopt this intervention.

Fig. 3.1 Systematic thinking for Evidence-based and Efficient Decision-making (SEED) tool.

3.2 Consideration Two

The second question underlines the need to have good-quality evidence on the effectiveness of any intervention. It is highly desirable that the evidence on intervention efficacy/effectiveness[2] should have been tested on the same (or at least very similar) population groups with the same dosage, frequency and other clinical and implementation characteristics — this homogeneity can reduce the risk of bias. There are many excellent appraisal tools for determining the quality of evidence. They are highlighted in an online resource called Enhancing the QUAlity and Transparency of Healthcare Research (EQUATOR) Network.[3] This online resource recommends different quality appraisal tools for different type of research. These include: the Consolidated Standards of Reporting Trials (CONSORT) for randomized control trials; the Preferred Reporting Items for Systematic Reviews and Meta-Analyses (PRISMA); the Strengthening the Reporting of Observational Studies in Epidemiology (STROBE); and the Consolidated Health Economic Evaluation Standards (CHEERS).

Alternatively, the quality of evidence on intervention effectiveness could be evaluated based on the hierarchy of evidence, which ranks different types of studies according to their 'academic rigor' (see Fig. 3.2 below and Chapter 7). In this pyramid, the evidence is strongest (lowest potential bias) for systematic reviews and meta-analyses of randomized control trials, followed by randomized control trials, cohort studies, case control studies and case series/reports (and some pyramids also include expert opinion below these other study designs). This hierarchy of evidence exists in various forms in the literature even though most of them have the same general format, with the validity and strength of the evidence based on the risk of bias (also called internal validity).[4] While it is helpful to use the hierarchy of evidence, it has limitations in

2 Efficacy = intervention performance under ideal and controlled circumstances; effectiveness = intervention performance under 'real-world' conditions.

3 Enhancing the QUAlity and Transparency Of Health Research (EQUATOR) Network, *The Strengthening the Reporting of Observational Studies in Epidemiology (STROBE) Statement: Guidelines for Reporting Observational Studies*, 2019, http://www.equator-network.org/reporting-guidelines/strobe/

4 Health Intervention and Technology Assessment Program (HITAP), *Guide to Health Economic Analysis and Research (GEAR) Online Resource: Guidelines Comparison*, 2019, http://www.gear4health.com/gear/health-economic-evaluation-guidelines

application, especially in LMICs where there is often a lack of quality data or resources to conduct more rigorous study designs.

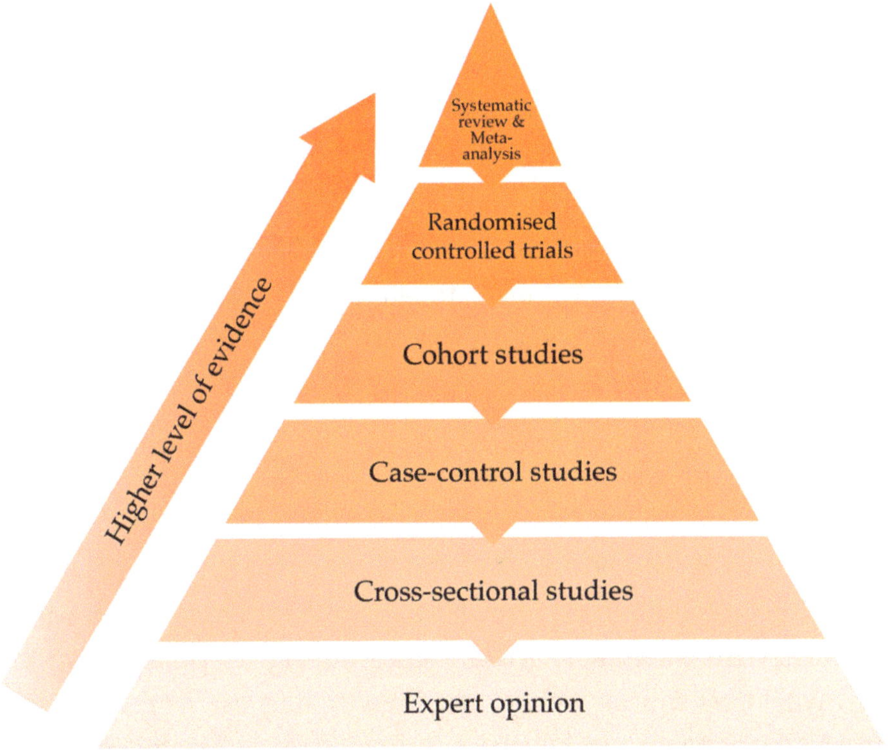

Fig. 3.2 Hierarchy of evidence. Source: Modified from New Evidence Pyramid.[5]

3.3 Consideration Three

The third question explores whether the studies' results can be applied to the population of interest and whether the intervention can be transferred to other settings (also called the external validity of the studies). This consideration requires examination of the external or contextual factors that may alter the effect of the intervention from the studies' settings to the implementation setting. This point is important since many countries (especially LMICs with limited resources for research) use evidence from other countries. An intervention with strong evidence from high-income countries might have less of an effect in more resource-constrained countries due to different population characteristics or a lack of supportive

5 M. Hassan Murad et al., 'New Evidence Pyramid', *Evidence Based Medicine*, 21.4 (2016), 125–27, https://doi.org/10.1136/ebmed-2016-110401; Health Intervention and Technology Assessment Program (HITAP).

factors (e.g., infrastructure or social norms). Even transferring the study results of an intervention within a country with vastly different regional contexts, such as applying the results of studies set in urban areas to sparsely populated remote areas, can change the intervention effect drastically. The local context, including environmental factors, should therefore always be considered for any studies used for policy-making. NCD managers and policymakers ought to scrutinize the evidence with professional care and ensure that the evidence is reasonably transferable to their context. If this is not the case, then investing in additional measures to address the potential changes in effect, such as training sessions, incentive structures, communications campaigns and awareness raising, should be considered.

3.4 Consideration Four

The fourth question addresses issues related to the cost of the intervention and its budget impact, i.e., cost-effectiveness, affordability and other cost outcomes. When considering a policy, especially preventive interventions where the health harvest is reaped in the future, NCD managers and decision-makers are confronted with higher early healthcare spending from the date of implementation onwards, whereas beneficial health outcomes will come later. Potential Best Buy interventions could be therefore be excluded from the NCD program. In this case, NCD managers should also consider how best to achieve the intervention within the budgetary constraints of the government or health provider; and, specifically to explore whether there are modifiable factors contributing to the high cost of the intervention, such as whether additional capital investment and human resource training will be needed and how they could affect the overall cost or the affordability. Governments, with the benefit of information provided from costing, cost-effectiveness, feasibility and budget impact studies can identify such factors, evaluate the long-term costs and benefits of the intervention and act to reduce the costs, thereby making them affordable and increasing the likelihood of a Best Buy.[6]

6 Adun Mohara et al., 'Using Health Technology Assessment for Informing Coverage Decisions in Thailand', *Journal of Comparative Effectiveness Research*, 1.2 (2012), 137–46, https://doi.org/10.2217/cer.12.10

3.5 Consideration Five

The last question asks whether there is political and professional support for the intervention in question. This consideration has different requirements compared to the previous questions, given that it is dependent on factors such as stakeholder consensus and buy-in, social and cultural influences and the governmental structure of the country. This issue is important because a Best Buy might be forgone if there is no political or professional support for it. 'Policy-informed evidence' might be deployed in response to high-level political pressures and influences instead of genuine evidence.[7] Managing this is tricky, but failure results in the implementation of suboptimal options, especially if this consideration is the first to be addressed in the SEED Tool (one reason for our recommendation to follow the logical order). For example, one of the case studies in this book discusses Thailand's implementation of a diabetes mellitus and hypertension screening program for the entire population, which was a good political investment even though there was a lack of evidence to support the policy fully.[8] An economic evaluation conducted later showed that targeted screening for high-risk groups was more cost-effective and led to a change in policy with the potential for reallocation of the budget to other NCD programs and a further improvement in health outcomes. This case was successful because of a commitment from all sectors. However, it is much better to ensure that policies are based on evidence from the outset and, where this is not established practice, to build a new culture in which it is expected. This implies making sure that professional and training institutions instill in students a clear understanding of evidence-informed decision-making processes and why they are important, and that the training of civil servants and other government officials and advisers likewise includes modules on evidence and decision-making.

7 Sarocha Chootipongchaivat et al., *Factors Conducive to the Development of Health Technology Assessment in Asia: Impacts and Policy Options* (Manila: World Health Organization, 2015), https://apps.who.int/iris/bitstream/handle/10665/208261/9789290617341_eng.pdf?sequence=1&isAllowed=y

8 See Chapter 5.

3.6 The SEED Tool in Practice

NCD prevention interventions are often complex and multi-faceted, requiring collective effort and time from both public and private players to implement. Consequently, they always come with a high opportunity cost for their introduction or maintenance within healthcare systems. The SEED Tool can be considered a framework or conceptualization that captures all necessary considerations to enhance the probability of implementing Best Buys and avoiding Wasted Buys. Each consideration in the tool has sub-considerations, which are discussed in other sections of this book — as such, the SEED Tool is the backbone of the book and the following chapters on Best Buys and Wasted Buys will illustrate the usefulness of applying it. This SEED Tool is also the starting point for in-depth discussion on technical and practical issues surrounding decision-making processes for health investment, such as the subjects of generalizability and transferability that will be described in Chapter 6 (see the Consideration 3 discussion above) and political buy-in, which is discussed in Chapter 2 as part of its illustration of the political economy of NCD prevention. Governance and process are covered in Chapter 9 (see the Consideration 5 discussion above).

The SEED Tool summarizes not only all the types of evidence — such as those produced in health technology assessments, health systems research, policy studies, etc. — it also incorporates contextual issues such as local intervention costs and political buy-in among key decision makers. Further, given the intricacies of NCD prevention interventions, there are many stakeholders within and outside the health sector with their own perspectives and areas of concern. Having a common framework in the SEED Tool that allows these relevant stakeholders to deliberate and/or prioritize all competing policy options can be crucial for the success of NCD prevention, which requires commitment and ownership at all levels of policy implementation.

This book benefits from using case studies to examine how NCD programs have been implemented in the past; this was an input in developing the SEED Tool. It is designed to be used for considering both new and existing interventions, whether it be for vertical programs or as part of broader public health systems. Specifically, the tool can be helpful in evaluating: 1) the impact of an existing program that will continue to be implemented, and exploring any changes necessary to improve the program; 2) a new program in consideration for implementation; 3) the effect of a program that was completed, to determine lessons learned; and, 4) an ongoing program for continuation. As such, it can be used to evaluate the impact of current or past programs retrospectively as well as to determine whether proposed interventions should be implemented in the future. The authors hope to use and also to test this framework, with the aim of avoiding Wasted Buys and increasing the likelihood of investing in Best Buys.

The tool has the potential to be applied not only for NCDs but also for other public health programs, or even as a system-wide mechanism for priority-setting (for example, as part of the inclusion of health technology or services in the benefits package or the essential medicines list). This tool can also be helpful when used together with priority-setting institutions and appropriate policy processes. This is because the authors believe that together evidence and process can be impactful, generating a loop of better evidence for better processes and vice versa, which eventually leads to better decisions with a greater impact on health.[9]

9 Rob Lloyd et al., *International Decision Support Initiative (IDSI) Theory of Change Review Report*', *F1000Research*, 7.1659 (2018).

4. Best Buys

Tazeem Bhatia, Arisa Shichijo and Ryota Nakamura

4.1 Introduction

4.1.1 Background

Because decision-makers need to prioritize policy options that bring the greatest possible health benefits from limited available resources, the World Health Organization (WHO) introduced Best Buys and other recommended cost-effective policy interventions to prevent and control NCDs.[1] The work, based on a rigorous process of review and selection, generated a menu of medical and public health interventions to reduce modifiable NCD risk factors in respect of diet, smoking, alcohol and physical activity, and to control and manage better the four major types of NCDs that contribute to 80% of global premature mortality from NCDs:[2] cardiovascular disease, diabetes, cancer and chronic respiratory disease, as summarized in Table 4.1.[3]

In addition to Best Buys, we also use the terms 'Wasted Buys' and 'Contestable Buys'. This chapter mainly covers Best Buys and Contestable

1 World Health Organization, *Tackling NCDs: Best Buys*, 2017, http://apps.who.int/iris/bitstream/handle/10665/259232/WHO-NMH-NVI-17.9-eng.pdf?sequence=1

2 World Health Organization, *Non-communicable Diseases: Key Facts 2018*, 2019, http://www.who.int/news-room/fact-sheets/detail/noncommunicable-diseases

3 World Health Organization, *Assessing National Capacity for the Prevention and Control of Noncommunicable Diseases*, ed. by Report of the 2017 Global Survey (Geneva: World Health Organization, 2017).

 https://doi.org/10.11647/OBP.0195.04

Table 4.1 WHO's list of Best Buys on NCD preventions.

Risk factor and diseases	Interventions
Tobacco use	• Tax increases
	• Plain/standardized packaging
	• Smoke-free workplaces and public places
	• Public awareness through mass media about the harms
	• Ban on tobacco advertising, promotion and sponsoring
Harmful alcohol use	• Tax increases
	• Restricted access to retailed alcohol
	• Bans on alcohol advertising
Unhealthy diet and physical inactivity	• Reduce salt intake in food through: ◊ Product reformulation ◊ Low salt options ◊ Food labelling ◊ Campaigns
	• Public awareness through mass media about physical activity
Cardiovascular disease and diabetes	• Counselling and multi-drug therapy (including glycemic and blood pressure control) for people with a high risk of developing cardiovascular events
Cancer	• Vaccination against human papillomavirus
	• Screening and treatment of pre-cancerous lesions to prevent cervical cancer

Buys.[4] An intervention is a Contestable Buy if there are only aspirations for, and hence no direct evidence of, cost-effectiveness in the country setting in which the intervention is being considered. Interventions in the WHO's Best Buys list may still be Contestable Buys if there is no demonstrative evidence of cost-effectiveness in the particular setting in question. The main distinction between Best and Contestable Buys is thus the availability of context-specific evidence. The reason why the distinction is important is that local context strongly influences the cost-effectiveness of an intervention.

4 See Chapter 5 for full discussion of Wasted Buys.

Data reviews confirm the scarcity of evidence of cost-effective Best Buys. Our analysis of the current evidence base in LMICs, based on the Global Health Cost Effectiveness Analysis Registry, identified very limited local evidence of Best Buys or of cost-effective preventive policies even for widely popular interventions such as taxation on tobacco and sugar-sweetened beverages (see Online Appendix 4A for an analysis of evidence by interventional type (Table 4A.1) and by country (Table 4A.2). We found country-specific evidence of Best Buy tobacco control policies in two countries only: Tanzania and Vietnam. Similarly, evidence of Best Buy alcohol control policies was found only in four relatively high-income countries: Australia, Denmark, Mexico and the Netherlands. Lack of local evidence creates uncertainty for decision-makers, who often have to rely on evidence transferred from other settings.[5]

A recent country capacity survey by WHO demonstrated that their list of Best Buys and other cost-effective interventions was 'underutilized' and that progress on NCDs globally was insufficient to meet 2030 goals.[6] There were many reasons for this, including but not limited to: 1) public health interventions are less likely than clinical interventions to have been subjected to cost-effective analyses for resource allocation decisions; 2) the evidence of the cost-effectiveness of those Best Buys as defined by the WHO report often does not come from their local decision context;[7] 3) a lack of adequate local capacity in implementing a Health Technology Assessment (HTA); 4) a limited awareness or demand for Cost-Effectiveness Analysis (CEA) from policy-makers in NCD prevention; and 5) the general absence of guidance either as to how to implement the recommended interventions on the Best Buys list or how to draw credible conclusions from the transfer of evidence between settings that have different disease burdens, different decision-making and managerial capacities, different institutional and

---

5 See Chapter 6 for assessing the transferability of economic evidence.

6 World Health Organization, *Assessing National Capacity for the Prevention and Control of Noncommunicable Diseases,* 2017, https://apps.who.int/iris/bitstream/handle/10665/276609/9789241514781-eng.pdf

7 Luke. N. Allen et al., 'Evaluation of Research on Interventions Aligned to WHO 'Best Buys' for NCDs in Low-Income and Lower-Middle-Income Countries: A Systematic Review from 1990 to 2015', *BMJ Global Health,* 3 (2018), e000535, https://doi.org/10.1136/bmjgh-2017-000535

delivery frameworks and different cultural and historical inheritances. Consequently, NCD policies are largely implemented without evidence of, or only with implicit assumptions about, cost-effectiveness.

4.1.2 What This Chapter Offers

Achieving Best Buy status largely depends on cost-effectiveness data, but there are many issues to settle if cost-effectiveness evidence is to be used for making decisions in real-world settings. These include the quality of the design and execution of the research on which the evidence is based, the extent to which cost and health outcomes observed elsewhere are likely to apply in a different context and the methodological challenges involved in comparing cost and health outcomes elsewhere with those of alternative interventions locally, as well as the practical challenges involved in introducing and sustaining the intervention. In this chapter we draw on real-world experiences in NCD policies and show how an intervention that is a Best Buy in ex-ante aspiration is compromised when implemented within a specific local context, turning it therefore into a Contestable Buy. This alteration is at least partly because real-world policies need to respond to the local context, such as culture, politics, history, market and law, within which they are implemented, and partly because of a common need to involve various stakeholders with vested interests who may be threatened by a novelty. There may also be important value judgements, such as judgements about equity, which might count in making decisions and which are locally specific. Furthermore, policies are not implemented in a vacuum but have synergistic and cumulative effects along with other policies, which in turn effect their potency. Prevention of NCDs is not just about addressing modifiable lifestyle risk factors but linking this to the social determinants of health, such as living and working environments, or economic policy and broader social policy.[8] We use the analysis of real-world case studies on NCD prevention to develop a list of considerations to help guide NCD managers and policy-makers through the design of the implementation process. This is not an alternative to the WHO's list of Best Buys, which can provide policy-makers with a useful starting point for planning NCD

8 See Chapter 2 for the discussion from the political aspect.

prevention interventions that potentially offer best value for money. The list is a secondary step to assist NCD managers in identifying a true local Best Buy and ensuring that it remains so during implementation, i.e., not remaining Contestable or even becoming Wasted.

To give an example of how local context can affect the impact and reach of an intervention, bike-sharing schemes, although not listed as a WHO Best Buy, are now popular in many countries, as they can encourage active commuting, hence physical activity,[9] as well as reducing congestion and potentially improving air quality. In Tehran, such a bike-sharing scheme is thriving, but only for men and not for women, due to the cultural and religious contexts that prevent women from taking part in the scheme.[10] This does not necessarily mean that the scheme in Tehran is a Wasted Buy. The scheme is successful, at least for men, and it may be deemed a Best Buy within this specific context. In this example, culture and religion are not modifiable factors, but need to be considered when making policy. There are other types of contextual factors that policy-makers can potentially modify, which are discussed in the following section.

4.2 Determining Important Contextual Factors in NCD Prevention

Why does context matter so much, which contextual factors matter most and how can we measure their effect?

Local contextual factors are often not subject to formal quantification in the same way as they are in cost-effectiveness analyses performed in high-income contexts. Real-world experiences are potentially useful and thought-provoking sources of information that can be used to identify which and how contextual factors interact with the implementation process. To gain some appreciation of real-world experience, we invited policy-makers and researchers from across the globe to share case studies of local implementations of NCD preventive policies. We

9 James Woodcock et al., 'Health Effects of the London Bicycle Sharing System: Health Impact Modelling Study', *BMJ*, 348 (2014), g425, https://doi.org/10.1136/bmj.g425

10 Russell Meddin, *Tehran's 'Bike House' Shines Green*, 2010, http://bike-sharing.blogspot.com/2010/03/tehrans-bike-house-shines-green.html

collected forty-seven case studies on the implementation of Best or Contestable Buys and summarize them in Table 4.2.[11]

Table 4.2 Summary of the collected case studies.

No. of case studies	Type of intervention	Country
Risk-factor prevention		
5	• Reduce tobacco use	India, Iran Philippines, Uganda
4	• Reduce the harmful use of alcohol and other substance misuse	Bhutan, Democratic Republic of the Congo, Philippines
1	• Reduce tobacco use & harmful use of alcohol	Kenya
12	• Reduce unhealthy diet	Bangladesh, Chile, China, Hungary, India, Iran, Philippines, South Africa, Zambia
2	• Increase physical activity	Bhutan, Rwanda
1	• Reduce unhealthy diet & increase physical activity	Haiti
Reduce disease through screening or immunization		
7	• Prevent diabetes or cardiovascular diseases	India, Kyrgyzstan, Philippines, Sri Lanka, Turkey, Uzbekistan
3	• Prevent cancer	Bangladesh, Cambodia, Honduras
5	**Improve health literacy**	Bangladesh, India, Philippines
1	**Increasing awareness and health literacy**	Indonesia
6	**Other — strengthen health system response**	Bangladesh, Iran, Ireland, Nepal, Slovenia

Although the forty-seven case studies do not necessarily represent successful NCD preventive policies, they provide useful insights into the reality of policy implementation. Twenty-five cases were specific to risk-factor modification: reducing tobacco use and sweetened beverage consumption were the most frequent. Ten cases were interventions to

11 See Online Appendix 4B for more detailed information and our analyses.

reduce disease through immunization or screening for risk or early disease. Six cases describe policies to increase public awareness and health literacy. The remaining six concerned strengthening the health system response to NCDs. We analyzed the case studies and then triangulated the findings with the existing literature on Best Buys and best practices in public health[12] to reveal factors that seem to be significant in the processes of policy formation and implementation in various contexts. The results are summarized in Table 4.3 and form a list of considerations. We propose that these considerations are used to supplement, but not to replace, cost-effectiveness when deciding whether and how to implement an NCD prevention intervention. We call them 'additional considerations' to emphasize that they are a supplementary step between the global list of NCD preventive policies and implementation in local settings, in order to ensure that a Best Buy when implemented is really a Best Buy — although this can be tested only through robust monitoring and evaluation.

In principle, whether an additional consideration is applicable is of course likely to be context-dependent, so what factors matter could differ by context. Although we applied the list of considerations to the forty-seven case studies as a score card (Online Appendix 4B), this list has not gone through the necessary testing to validate it as a tool, a quantitative measure, or a score for each of the considerations. At this stage, it is a summary of wisdom drawn from real-world experiences, or a set of prompts or questions to ask when implementing and evaluating NCD preventive policies — hence why we call them considerations and not prerequisite steps. Likewise, the list is not a checkbox tool to identify a Best Buy that substitutes for local evidence of cost-effectiveness. Rather, the list should be used to assess proposed interventions and predict critical stumbling blocks that stem from local contexts, in particular when there is a desire to acquire a particular Best Buy, but its suitability needs testing. The considerations can be used to complement the SEED Tool (in particular consideration 3, 4 and 5) in Chapter 3, to give the intervention a better chance of being a Best Buy in the specific context of its possible implementation.

12 Eileen Ng and Pierpaolo de Colombani, 'Framework for Selecting Best Practices in Public Health: A Systematic Literature Review', *Journal of Public Health Research*, 4.3 (2015), https://doi.org/10.4081/jphr.2015.577

Table 4.3 Additional considerations for making and judging Best Buy NCD preventive policies.

Category	Question to ask yourself	Common issues for consideration	Number of case studies
Relevance	Is the prevention intervention relevant to this community?	• Prevalence and burden of NCD	41/47
		• Policy-makers' awareness and knowledge	40/47
		• Priority of NCD in health system	24/47
		• Culture, tradition, convention and norm e.g., Religion, ethnicity, popularity of unhealthy behavior	23/47
		• Acceptability and consumer demand	11/47
		• Other existing interventions to tackle this problem	17/47
Leadership, governance, compliance	Will I be supported to implement the intervention? Will the legislation be enforced?	• Political mandate and stability to tackle NCD	32/47
		• Conflict of interest e.g., Industry opposition	17/47
		• System and market structure e.g., Market structure is too complex to design interventions	21/47
		• Enforcement of legislation locally e.g., Smuggling, black market	21/47
		• Transparency and accountability e.g., Held to account by civil society	21/47

Table 4.3 (continued) Additional considerations for making and judging Best Buy NCD preventive policies.

Category	Question to ask yourself	Common issues for consideration	Number of case studies
Sustainability	Will the intervention be sustainably implemented?	• Funding and affordability	22/47
		• Human resources and skills	22/47
		• Infrastructure, facility and equipment	23/47
		• Integration of NCD prevention into health system e.g., Practical guidelines, monitoring system	18/47
		• Local ownership	15/47
Multisectoral collaboration	Who should I collaborate with and how? Who are the stakeholders who will make this happen?	• Implementation as part of non-health policy e.g., Tax policy, bike share	16/47
		• Motivation and incentive	15/47
		• Networking and power dynamic among stakeholders	21/47
		• Overlapping priorities among ministries	13/47
Community and stakeholder involvement	Will the community engage? Will my intervention reach my target population?	• Community engagement	28/47
		• Community's access to NCD prevention programs e.g., Scaling up an intervention to a wider population	27/47
		• Community and organizational capacity e.g., Health literacy	18/47
Ethics and values	Is it ethically acceptable to implement the intervention?	• Health equity and effect on health inequalities	13/47
		• (Re)distribution of burden	6/47
	What might be the unintended consequences of this action or externalities?	• Economic side effects e.g., Unemployment	4/47
		• Ethical permission	2/47

4.3 Policymaking Challenges and Cost-Effectiveness Data

In this section, we apply cost-effectiveness and the additional considerations in Table 4.3 as a score card to assess policies for NCD prevention in LMICs and highlight those contextual factors that are critical; we also set out why and how these contextual factors make the implementation of NCD preventive policies complicated and challenging.

When the set of questions in Table 4.3 was applied to the forty-seven case studies submitted by policy-makers and researchers,[13] the most striking finding was that in the real world many of the Best Buys became Contestable Buys because of the nature of the evidence and implementation issues within the specific context. We give examples of this below. In fact, only three out of the forty-seven cases were explicitly informed by local cost-effectiveness data, suggesting that such data are probably rarely available and highly unlikely to be used by policy-makers in the decision-making process. We hypothesized in the introduction that cost-effectiveness evidence alone was in any case insufficient to determine which interventions should be prioritized and indicated the other considerations that might apply. This set of case studies suggests that cost-effectiveness evidence is rarely used to prioritize interventions. Further, fewer than half of the cases (seventeen out of forty-seven) were even informed by local data on effectiveness. Table 4.3 (fourth column) shows the number of case studies that mentioned each consideration, as judged by the chapter authors. The local relevance of NCDs was addressed in most of the case studies. They described the burden of disease, its magnitude and the awareness of the problem, but fewer than half the cases described the relevance of the chosen intervention in terms of the local culture, traditions and behavior, or in relation to other interventions already being implemented. Only half of the case studies explored the potential acceptability of their proposed approaches or the sustainability of the intervention in terms of financial or human resources. The case studies that described the implementation of a fiscal measure, for example taxation on tobacco or on sugar-sweetened beverages, particularly emphasized the importance

13 See Online Appendix 4B.

of political economy issues, including industry and other stakeholders' opposition to implementation.

The literature discusses the importance of effective public engagement and the need to ensure equitable representation of all groups in the composition of participation. Health equity and distributional justice are offered as critical issues given that an approach that seeks to maximize health benefits for a population can conflict with efforts to achieve equity.[14] Despite this, community engagement or health equity were rarely considered or explicitly mentioned in our cases.

4.4 Investigating Case Studies

The case studies gave a rich description of contextual challenges and enablers. We feature and investigate the forty-seven case studies[15] and share examples of NCD prevention policies that faced challenges in implementation.

Case Study 4.4.1 Cardiovascular screening in Sri Lanka[16]

Sri Lanka is estimated to have the highest death rates due to NCDs in South Asia[17], with many patients presenting late in the disease progression. A national survey reported that 36% of all patients with diabetes were undetected.[18] In response, the government formulated a National Policy and Strategic Framework for prevention and control of chronic non-communicable disease which included implementation of a CVD risk screening program at community level.[19] This policy was implemented nationally through the establishment of 'Healthy

14 Ng and Colombani.

15 In Appendix 4B you can see the detailed analysis of the forty-seven case studies.

16 Authors of this case study: Rohan Jayasuriya (University of New South Wales, Australia), Sumudu Karunaratne (Ministry of Health, Sri Lanka) and Amala de Silva (University of Colombo, Sri Lanka).

17 World Health Organization, 'Global Health Estimates 2016: Deaths by Cause, Age, Sex, by Country and by Region, 2000-2016' (Geneva: World Health Organization, 2016).

18 Prasad Katulanda et al., 'Prevalence and Projections of Diabetes and Pre-Diabetes in Adults in Sri Lanka-Sri Lanka Diabetes, Cardiovascular Study (SLDCS)', *Diabetic Medicine*, 25.9 (2008), 1062–69, https://doi.org/10.1111/j.1464-5491.2008.02523.x

19 Ministry of Healthcare and Nutrition Sri Lanka, *The National Policy & Strategic Frame Work for Prevention and Control of Chronic Non- Communicable Diseases*, 2009, http://www.health.gov.lk/enWeb/publication/Act/NCDPolicy-English.pdf

Lifestyle Clinics' (HLCs) in 2011, initially funded by the World Bank. At present, there are 800 HLCs functioning in Sri Lanka.[20] Several pilot studies informed the decision including the NCD Prevention Project (NPP), which was funded by the Japan International Corporation Agency.[21] The NPP study tested two approaches. Both approaches had similar criteria for inclusion, all individuals between 40–75 years of age, without a history of NCDs. The first approach (a two-step model) involved screening by body mass index and blood pressure in the community and then diagnostic testing (fasting capillary glucose and blood pressure) in a health clinic. The second approach (a one-step model) implemented screening and diagnostic testing at the same time in hospital. They achieved similar detection rates for risk factors including high blood pressure and diabetes and coverage of population. However, the two-step model saw a significantly higher follow-up rate of 85%, compared to 19% in the one-step model, which is a crucial finding as chronic disease management resulting in glycaemic control and control of hypertension in moderately high-risk individuals is the motivation for screening. In the two-step model, the field staff (Public Health Midwives — PHMs) were able to trace those who were at risk, resulting in higher follow up. However, neither model evaluated the cost-effectiveness of the approaches. Policy makers felt unable to justify implementing the two-step model in the national rollout due to issues of feasibility (affordability, health system structure and workforce capacity). The PHMs could not be deployed on a national level as it would distract from their core midwifery functions. Donors and policy-makers therefore backed the expansion of the one-step model through HLC, accepting that compromises in implementation are often necessary.

The case study from Sri Lanka, featured in the box, describes one of the pilot studies undertaken and the review of evidence generated prior to designing a National Cardiovascular (CVD) Screening program. If they

20 D.S. Virginie Mallawaarachchi et al., 'Healthy Lifestyle Centres: A Service for Screening Non-communicable Diseases through Primary Health-Care Institutions in Sri Lanka', *WHO South-East Asia Journal of Public Health*, 5.2 (2016), 89, https://doi.org/10.4103/2224-3151.206258

21 Japan International Cooperation Agency, *Project on Health Promotion and Preventice Care Measures of Chronic NCDs Final Report* (Tokyo: Japan International Corporation Agency, 2013), http://open_jicareport.jica.go.jp/pdf/12112322.pdf

had applied the list of additional considerations, Sri Lanka could have ticked many of the boxes. Relevance was established, local evidence was generated and political will and donor support were critical to realizing and determining the contents of this national program. Inadequate local capacity, however, became a stumbling block to implementing the preferred model of delivery. Evidence suggests that drug treatment for those at high risk of CVD (total risk of CVD event >30%) is a cost-effective intervention and a Best Buy,[22] so by choosing the approach that yielded fewer follow-up visits and therefore chronic disease management the Sri Lankans may have undermined the effectiveness and cost-effectiveness of this program. Compromise and pragmatism are often required in the real world, but the consequences of decisions need to be captured. An evaluation of the program should capture not only the percentage of the eligible population that has been screened and identify modifiable risk factors like smoking and hypertension, but also outcomes such as the number of patients with controlled hypertension. This is a way of measuring the impact of the program as currently structured. The results may point to some constraints that could be easily addressed. For example, a recent review of the routine data for this CVD risk screening program showed that more than two thirds of the attendees were women. It was quickly realized that this was because the screening occurs during the official working week, i.e., Monday to Friday, which was preventing men from benefiting from the scheme and resulting in a rectifiable inequity. The Public Health Midwives or other primary health staff, as well as community representatives, should be invited to contribute to finding a solution for the workforce capacity issues and community participation in the screening program. Local areas may want to pilot different solutions.

Case Study 4.4.2 Prevention and control of cervical cancer in Cambodia

Another case study, authored by Koum Kanal, concerned prevention and control of cervical cancer in Cambodia. Cervical cancer in Cambodia is one of the most serious yet preventable health problems. Cambodia implemented a pilot study of a new cervical cancer program, which was

22 World Health Organization, *Tackling NCDs: Best Buys.*

based on the WHO's guide to Comprehensive Cervical Cancer Control.[23] The program aimed to: 1) raise access to cervical cancer screening among factory workers; 2) improve gynecologic capacity for diagnosis and treatment of precancerous lesions; and 3) strengthen pathological capacity for cancer diagnosis. The implementation was supported by strong political will and involved ministries and donors, which facilitated international collaborations of professional associations. The cost of the new screening program was estimated to be less than 1 US dollar per person per year and was therefore financially sustainable. Although there is no direct cost-effectiveness evidence, the program was likely to be highly cost-effective and hence a Best Buy. However, the most striking barrier to nationwide implementation was again an inadequate local capacity to scale up the program nationally — there were only four pathologists in the country and built infrastructure was also needed. Cambodia started a new pathology residency program in the country in 2015, in which five residents are trained with support from Japanese and German universities. A technician-capacity-building program was also initiated. While these capacities are being developed, temporary measures could be explored and, wherever affordable, adopted to meet the needs of the screening and management, including outsourcing; e.g., contracting a pathology service with neighborhood countries or requesting international co-operation, which means setting up a program and guidelines for pathologists from outside of the country to effectively work in the Cambodian context with limited human resources and skills.

Case Study 4.4.3 Sugar-Sweetened Beverage (SSB) taxes

The SSB tax to discourage sugar consumption is probably the approach currently being most tested, partly because of the popularity of SSBs across cultures, the worldwide increase in sales and their price-sensitivity, especially in low and low-middle-income countries.[24] South

23 World Health Organization, *Comprehensive Cervical Cancer Control: A Guide to Essential Practic* (WHO Library Cataloguing-in-Publication Data, 2014), https://apps.who.int/iris/bitstream/handle/10665/144785/9789241548953_eng.pdf?sequence=1

24 Yevgeniy Goryakin et al., 'Soft Drink Prices, Sales, Body Mass Index and Diabetes: Evidence from a Panel of Low-, Middle- and High-Income Countries', *Food Policy*, 73 (2017), 88–94, https://doi.org/10.1016/j.foodpol.2017.09.002

Africa, Zambia, Chile and Philippines all submitted case studies on SSB taxation (authored by Karen Hofman, Surgey et al., Cristóbal Cuadrado, Frances Claire Onagan, respectively). They described the policy process and the challenges faced when implementing an effective tax to improve health, as well as how the impact of these additional considerations can affect whether the intervention is a Best Buy for health or not.

SSB taxes are notably announced and led by Ministries of Finance (MoF) or Health (MoH) or in some instances by the Head of State and thus are a classic example of a multisectoral approach. When implementing SSB taxes, the MoF's primary objective is not necessarily health improvement, but revenue creation. Implementation of an SSB tax tends to be subject to strong opposition by industry, which tries to limit its impact. Even when there is strong political leadership in tackling NCDs, such special interests can have implications for the level at which taxes are set and this is a challenge for the health sector. In many countries, SSB tax rates are moderate (for example at 5%), which may not significantly influence consumer purchasing in the long run, in which case the tax serves only as a revenue-raising mechanism.[25] For example, Zambia is proposing a 3% tax that modelling has shown to have no benefit on health, but which will raise about $33,314 USD per annum in revenue. For the authors of this chapter, the Zambia SSB tax would be a Contestable Buy as it is unable to demonstrate health benefit, but it is not a Wasted Buy as it generates government revenue that could be used to fund other preventive or treatment interventions — hence the tax policy can be part of a Best Buy policy package and creates awareness of the risk of SSB consumption among the public which can lead to behavioral change.

These case studies highlight the importance of conflict of interest and of taking account of the resulting powerful influence of industry in creating doubt, determining the rate of the tax and on mediating the impact of taxation on consumers, thus weakening the political will for action. They underline the importance of engaging with the public, the need for strong advocacy, the value of local evidence and the importance of publicly countering industry arguments. Where taxes have been implemented without strong public health messaging to encourage

25 World Health Organization, *Using Price Policies to Promote Healthier Diets. Copenhagen: WHO Regional Office for Europe*, 2015, http://www.euro.who.int/__data/assets/pdf_file/0008/273662/Using-price-policies-to-promote-healthier-diets.pdf

consumer demand for healthier products, populations have interpreted the policy action as governments finding another way to extract money from them, which makes the intervention less acceptable to the public.[26]

4.5 Discussion

We endorse the WHO Best Buys for tackling NCDs but recommend that NCD decision-makers use local, context-specific cost-effectiveness information where obtainable, as well as the additional considerations, to prioritize interventions and to undertake the effective implementation of their chosen intervention. The Best Buy list is a list of evidenced interventions that have been shown to be cost-effective in more than one setting. The list contains interventions that are indeed Best Buys in some places and times and it provides a strong resource for countries to draw on. Unfortunately, there is no 'one size fits all' and the user of the list should not generalize and passively expect the interventions to be cost-effective in their setting just because they were in another; instead they should actively enquire whether the intervention is likely actually to be cost-effective in their setting. The user should assess any additional considerations that are of local relevance, given their specific country with its own constraints (budgetary and other), values, institutions and capacities. Users should also appreciate that contexts will require a different combination of policies to address a health challenge, that an intervention on its own might not be cost- effective, but in combination with others might form a cost-effective package.

We have proposed a list of considerations for assessing the possible importance of locally contextual, additional considerations, covering relevant areas including: culture, religion and ethnicity; leadership, governance and compliance; sustainability; multisectoral collaboration; community and stakeholder involvement; ethics and values (Table 4.3). The case studies have demonstrated that, in the real world, compromises are often made in the implementation process.

As a policy-maker, adviser or NCD manager using this list of additional considerations in your planning process, what do you

26 Orly Tamir et al., 'Taxation of Sugar Sweetened Beverages and Unhealthy Foods: A Qualitative Study of Key Opinion Leaders' Views', *Israel Journal of Health Policy Research*, 7.1 (2018), 43, https://doi.org/10.1186/s13584-018-0240-1

do if there are unsatisfactory answers to some of questions posed in Table 4.3? How do you explore whether the consequence of these considerations is sufficiently serious to reject the proposed intervention or whether it is possible to take complementary steps to mitigate the consequences? One solution could be to conduct a workshop and/or set up an advisory group with experts and policy-makers to explore the issues and any potential controversies, and design the necessary monitoring and measurement programs for an evaluation. Constraints (especially political and professional ones) could be overcome in several ways, for example: through price negotiations to increase affordability of the more effective model; investment in training and human capital to strengthen the sustainability and infrastructure elements; involving a wider range of public and private stakeholders from other governmental departments, the universities, professions and industry; and facing up to ethical and cultural challenges, for example, by encouraging open public debate on the critical issues.

Sometimes a Buy may be deemed to be Contestable on the grounds of the quality of the evidence. This is not usually a matter of local context.[27] The problem will often lie in the design of the primary research or in the reviews and meta-analyses that underlie the case, or in the data used, which may raise significant questions of transferability. Again, one way forward might be to conduct workshops of experts and policy-makers at which the issues and possible solutions and compromises can be explored. The forty-seven case studies demonstrated that little local evidence of effectiveness or cost-effectiveness is currently being utilized, probably because it is not available, but possibly also because of a lack of awareness that workable tools exist. Therefore, another possibility might be to conduct further research to address data deficiencies either at a local level or regionally, to incorporate other criteria than cost-effectiveness alone in the evaluation of the intervention in question and, in general, to raise awareness that will have consequential implications for training. All these will raise further questions of timing and funding.

In all cases good judgment is called for, which underlines the importance of regarding cost-effectiveness analysis and related methods as aids to thought rather than substitutes for it. It is important for decision-makers to understand the basics of the evaluative methodologies

27 See Chapter 7.

involved and their limitations, so that they can interrogate both the evidence and the experts intelligently and reach sound conclusions about the design and operation of the decision-making processes used in the country.

Best Buys are not necessarily 'quick fixes'. Modelling their return on investment involves projections over two to three decades. The fact that benefits from NCD prevention policies and interventions might not be felt until way into the future makes them politically difficult to justify, especially when the benefits accrue to one government department, but the spend falls on another. A significant number of the Best Buy policies need to be implemented by other sectors or with other sectors.[28] Even in the case of the revenue-generating fiscal policies where the costs of implementation and monitoring could be covered by the revenue generated, it was acknowledged that there were challenges with enforcing legislation or guidance.

Policy-makers need to balance national spending priorities fairly and efficiently while at the same time safeguarding an individual's right to health. Achieving equity can be costlier as it means reaching less accessible, often marginalized groups, thus potentially deeming the intervention, or some aspects of it, cost-ineffective. This emphasizes one of the challenges of applying CEA tools to public health interventions. Public health interventions are often more concerned with the distribution of health gains rather than maximizing health benefits or efficiency. The current economic evaluation methodology almost exclusively concerns the latter. In addition, due to the broad nature of the costs and benefits incurred, economists need an intersectoral approach to identify them and to measure health and social gain (see Chapter 8 on cross-sectoral policies to address NCDs). For example, a DALY may not be broad enough to identify all the benefits to society.[29]

4.6 Conclusion

In this chapter, we have made the case that cost-effectiveness data are generally scarce in NCD prevention in LMICs and that available data are

28 See Chapter 8 for cross-sectoral policies to address NCDs.

29 Helen Weatherly et al., 'Methods for Measuring Cost Effectiveness of Public Health Interventions: Key Challenges and Recommendations', *Health Policy*, 93.2–3 (2009), 85–92, https://doi.org/10.1016/j.healthpol.2009.07.012

not always generalizable to different settings. A crucial element of cost-effectiveness analysis is context sensitivity, meaning that a list of Best Buys generated at a global level cannot be assumed to be a Best Buy in a local setting unless there is local evidence of cost-effectiveness. Through a series of case study examples, we have sought to demonstrate the importance of context and developed a list of considerations in policy implementation to help NCD managers to judge whether a potential Best Buy intervention is effective and cost-effective in their own setting. In order to strengthen the effectiveness and cost-effectiveness of NCD prevention interventions, funders, national governments and technical agencies should consider investing in the following:

1. Regional support units to assist in the generation of regional and local cost-effectiveness evidence with local academics and health economists. This collaboration can enable the sharing of experiences and insights both in implementing NCD preventive policies and conducting HTAs, and also build the capacities of junior researchers and policy-makers through experiences and knowledge exchanges.[30]
2. Prioritization and decision-making processes that are informed by cost-effectiveness evidence such as the Lancet NCDI (non-communicable diseases and injuries) Commission[31], which familiarizes NCD managers and policy-makers with cost-effectiveness data and tools. This should increase the demand for such information and, hence, its production.
3. Development of further tools to assist in implementation. The list of additional considerations is a starting point for guiding managers and policy-makers. Further efforts should be invested in designing and validating a tool that is user friendly with a quantitative measure and/or composite score. Tools such as the tobacco control playbook developed by WHO Europe, which supports NCD managers and policy-makers with evidence-based arguments to defend tobacco control

30 Yot Teerawattananon et al., 'Historical Development of the HTAsiaLink Network and Its Key Determinants of Success', *International Journal of Technology Assessment in Health Care*, 34.3 (2018), 260–66, https://doi.org/10.1017/s0266462318000223

31 Gene Bukhman et al., 'Reframing NCDs and Injuries for the Poorest Billion: A Lancet Commission', *The Lancet*, 386.10000 (2015), 1221–22, https://doi.org/10.1016/s0140-6736(15)00278-0

policies in parliament, are useful guidance documents in that they prevent the weakening and subsequent ineffectiveness of such policies,[32] but offer no assessment of the implementation process. Academics are currently working to develop a tool to explicitly incorporate the notion of context when implementing public policies, which could be used to steer this process.[33]

4. Monitoring and evaluation of existing NCD prevention policies and interventions with a view to strengthening implementation and impact.
5. Best practice pilots that can generate further evidence of implementation methods and pitfalls.

32 World Health Organization, *Tobacco Control Playbook*, 2019, http://www.euro.who.int/en/health-topics/disease-prevention/tobacco/policy/tobacco-control-playbook

33 Politics and Ideas, *Context Matters: A Framework to Support Knowledge into Policy*, 2016, http://cm.politicsandideas.org/homepage

5. Wasted Buys

Yot Teerawattananon, Manushi Sharma, Alia Luz, Waranya Rattanavipapong and Adam G. Elshaug

5.1 Introduction

In 2011, approximately 6.9 trillion USD were spent globally on health, of which 20–40% were thought by the WHO to be wasted.[1] This evidence is corroborated by the Organization for Economic Co-operation and Development (OECD), which found that potentially one-fifth of total health spending in developed countries is wasted.[2] This observation is an example of inefficiency, and waste on this scale is far more serious in LMICs, where the overall burden of disease is so much higher and relatively small expenditures can have enormous impact (if spent wisely). The usual methods of controlling rising health expenditures have been either through structural reorganization or cost-cutting measures. The former is time-consuming and carries risks of missing the intended mark, an approach famously lampooned by Maynard in the UK as 'redisorganization',[3] while the latter is a blunt instrument and may impinge indiscriminately on both cost-effective and cost-ineffective parts of the system. Often the missing piece of this conundrum is figuring out how to eliminate waste and/or low-value health care. Efficiency gains from measures to improve health outcomes can be dispersed across sectors, but also have the potential to allow reallocation from poor value, low-impact interventions to

1 World Health Organization, *Global Health Expenditure Atlas* (Geneva: WHO Press, 2014), https://www.who.int/health-accounts/atlas2014.pdf

2 OECD, *Tackling Wasteful Spending on Health*, 2017, https://www.oecd.org/health/tackling-wasteful-spending-on-health-9789264266414-en.htm

3 Alan Maynard, 'What about Value for Money?', *BMJ*, 342 (2011), https://doi.org/10.1136/bmj.d1319

 https://doi.org/10.11647/OBP.0195.05

high-value, high-impact ones: a rare win-win for healthcare. Low-value resource allocation exists for a multitude of reasons: lack of evidence needed to create better health outcomes or to identify cheaper but equally effective procedures; poor management and weak coordination; social and political factors that may be of little general benefit to the community; the knowledge deficits and biases of the policy-makers and program managers; and governance-related waste such as fraud and corruption.[4]

This problem of low-value care is increasingly recognized in clinical medicine.[5] Many countries are now promoting the use of generic medicines,[6] seeking to prevent unnecessary interventions, avoiding adverse events and improving the targeting of tests and interventions to those most likely to benefit. However, much less is known about inefficient spending on the prevention and control of non-communicable diseases (NCDs) at the programmatic level. This chapter aims to fill this gap.

Our objective is to show that tackling inefficient spending or 'Wasted Buys' is a value-enhancing agenda which acts as a catalyzer in achieving the ultimate goals of a healthcare system. We provide an operational, pragmatic definition of Wasted Buys which will help program managers and policy-makers to identify inefficient spending and initiate a constructive dialogue; explain the common characteristics of inefficient spending incurred in the prevention of NCDs with current examples; and show how inefficient spending can be avoided by substituting better care at the same cost, more efficient care (more benefit compared to incremental cost), or cheaper alternatives with the same or even better health outcomes.

5.1.1 What Are 'Wasted Buys'?

The scalability of any intervention is subject to available evidence, which is often lacking, or is of variable quality, or is not context specific. What constitutes waste is often revealed in an implementation setting that is different from the study setting that generated the existing evidence, so

4 Vikas Saini et al., 'Addressing Overuse and Underuse around the World', *The Lancet*, 390 (2017), 105–7, https://doi.org/10.1016/S0140-6736(16)32573-9

5 Shannon Brownlee et al., 'Evidence for Overuse of Medical Services around the World', *The Lancet*, 390 (2017), 156–68, https://doi.org/10.1016/S0140-6736(16)32585-5

6 OECD, 'Pharmaceutical Spending Trends and Future Challenges', in *Health at*

that what might be seen as wasted in one context might not be wasted in another. So how should a program manager identify a Wasted Buy?

The OECD defines 'waste' in a developed country context as: (i) services and processes that are either harmful or do not deliver benefits; and (ii) costs that could be avoided by substituting cheaper alternatives with identical or better benefits.[7] Developed countries have well-established priority-setting mechanisms and data capture, which can be synthesized into relevant evidence to guide health policy. Developing countries pose a range of challenges in conducting a cost-effectiveness analysis, such as interpreting the poor-quality or non-contextual data used to estimate costs and effects, the choice of the comparator and whether subgroups of the target population are analyzed. There are therefore many uncertainties about how best to proceed. A comprehensive, pragmatic definition that fits the LMIC context is therefore required.

Recalling the analysis of Chapter 1, we treat Wasted Buys as interventions that fall in the shaded area in Figure 5.1, while interventions falling in Section 2 of Quadrant B and the whole of Quadrant D are not Wasted Buys.

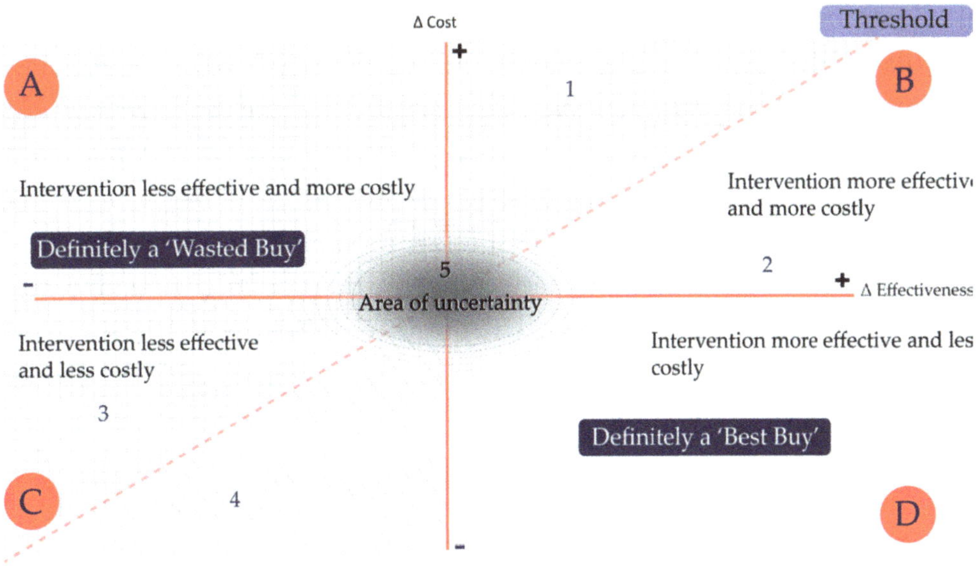

Fig. 5.1 Wasted Buys on a cost-effectiveness plane.

a Glance 2015 (Paris: OECD Publishing, 2015), https://www.google.com/search?q=Pharmaceutical+Spending+Trends+and+Future+Challenges&oq=Pharmaceutical+Spending+Trends+and+Future+Challenges&aqs=chrome..69i57j0.831j0j4&sourceid=chrome&ie=UTF-8

7 OECD, *Tackling Wasteful Spending on Health.*

Wasted Buys include interventions that deliver no health benefits (Quadrant A); interventions that yield a higher cost per unit of health outcome gained than the cost-effectiveness threshold in that setting (Section 1 of Quadrant B); and interventions that have low efficacy or no significant positive impact on health outcomes albeit at a meagre cost (Section 3 in Quadrant C). Interventions falling in Section 4 in Quadrant C may need to be deliberated. For instance, interventions with a negative impact may be Contestable or even Best Buys if the cost reduction is sufficiently large to enable more health benefits to be gained elsewhere. Lastly, interventions that have a small cost or benefit impact, or about which there is substantial uncertainty, which fall in the 'area of uncertainty' should be carefully scrutinized before implementation (Section 5).

5.1.2 The 'Area of Uncertainty'

The area of uncertainty (Section 5) has a fuzzy boundary. It has no sharp edges. The area of uncertainty includes interventions that have substantially uncertain benefits or cost-effectiveness. There are three reasons for this. The first is a lack of knowledge and information about the benefits and/or costs of an intervention, as when an intervention is still in the experimental phase or implemented with insufficient understanding of the context. The second is uncertainty around estimations of effect, cost and cost-effectiveness that may come from parameter uncertainty, model uncertainty and uncertainties concerning the assumptions used — for example, in modelling future streams of benefit beyond experimental periods, or in the use of a constant rate of disease incidence over time. Uncertainty afflicts both clinical and economic studies. Finally, generalizability issues occur with proposals to implement an intervention in a new setting with conditions that vary from the study setting.

It is plainly important to note whether the radius of the circle is large or small or, indeed, whether it is a circle. This might remain unknown until further research has been conducted. The importance of understanding these different aspects of uncertainty may also vary across interventions, depending on several factors, such as the infeasibility of some interventions in resource-limited settings. While the cost-effectiveness plane is useful in understanding the types of uncertainty that affect cost, benefit and cost-effectiveness, it does not account for the uncertainties that are unrelated to ex-ante evaluations (conducted prior to the implementation), such as those implicit in the implementation of the intervention itself.

5.2 Exploring Wasted Buys in Low- and Middle-Income Countries (LMICs)

While Best Buys are recognized and widely acknowledged, the existence of Wasted Buys and even Contestable Buys has only just started to gain traction in the health community. The concept of Wasted Buys is broad and examples abound in many countries. To better understand the nature of Wasted Buys, we reviewed the literature to identify studies that illustrated ineffective and cost-ineffective interventions. The review focused on economic evaluations of preventive interventions in non-communicable diseases. We searched the Cochrane Collaboration Database, the Global Health Cost-Effectiveness Analysis (GH CEA) Registry from the Tufts Medical Center and the Disease Control Priorities project.

A. Cochrane Collaboration Database

Effectiveness is a necessary (but not sufficient) starting point to ensure the benefits of an intervention for the health system or to identify a Best Buy. If an ineffective intervention has been implemented, it counts as a low value or a 'Wasted Buy'. The Cochrane Collaboration database[8] is a trustworthy resource and has curated content on the effectiveness of a variety of interventions. We reviewed interventions focusing on negative or inconclusive results. Cochrane reviews related to mass-media campaigns for NCD preventions were selected and are discussed in detail in the next section.

8 'Cochrane | Trusted Evidence. Informed Decisions. Better Health', 2019, https://www.cochrane.org/

B. The Global Health Cost-Effectiveness Analysis (GH CEA) Registry

We reviewed articles from the GH CEA Registry[9] to establish the usefulness of the database and to understand the 'cost-per-DALY averted' approach to identifying Wasted Buy interventions. The review covered research conducted in LMICs; research on four specific NCDs: cancer, cardiovascular diseases (CVD), chronic respiratory diseases and diabetes; and intervention(s) for NCD prevention. Interventions were classified as Wasted Buys if the ICER was greater than three times the gross domestic product (GDP) per capita (which is referred to as a proxy for decision-making in LMICs that lack local research on thresholds) or if the ICER was negative, meaning that the intervention is costlier and less effective than the comparator(s). Nine studies were identified, of which one, a study on the cost-effectiveness of medical primary prevention strategies to reduce absolute risk of cardiovascular disease in Tanzania, was selected for review in detail.

C. Disease Control Priorities (DCP)

The three editions of the DCP that have been published focus on cost-effective options according to current research: they highlight potential Best Buys, or interventions that yield the most benefits in terms of health outcomes compared to cost. We reviewed the DCP's second edition and selected sections of the third to assess the project's ability to shed light on Wasted Buys as well as Contestable Buys and Best Buys. The following chapters of DCP II were selected: Health Service Interventions for Cancer Control in Developing Countries; Diabetes: The Pandemic and Potential Solutions; Cardiovascular Disease; and Respiratory Diseases in Adults. From DCP III, Volume 3 (Cancer) and Volume 5 (Cardiovascular, Respiratory and Related Disorders) were selected. The DCP authors conducted systematic reviews of high-burden diseases and economic evaluations, including diabetes in developing countries. They explored the interventions that

---

9 Center for the Evaluation of Value and Risk in Health (CEVR) Tufts Medical Center, 'Global Health CEA Registry', 2019, http://healtheconomics.tuftsmedicalcenter.org/ghcearegistry/

were mentioned as being of lower priority due to cost-ineffectiveness, less clinical benefit, infeasibility and other relevant considerations. They are non-prescriptive and were published without the use of any specific threshold or willingness to pay for an intervention. In addition, many of the studies used different methods and had no standard outcome measures. Since performance of the interventions in the implementation setting is a major consideration in identifying Best or Wasted Buys, interventions from the DCP project require further study or research for their transferability across settings.[10]

To analyze context-specific factors that might lead to Wasted Buys and that capture the perspective of program managers, we placed a call for case studies (as described in Chapter 1). This was circulated through a variety of networks. Fifty-eight case studies from thirty countries were received. Case studies that were deemed relevant to the NCDs theme were then analyzed (see Online Appendix 4B). A considerable portion of the cases submitted as Best Buys were not based on any evidence other than international guidelines or other countries' precedents. This is reflected in the case studies on diabetes screening in Indonesia and Thailand and drug testing among civil servants in Bhutan.

Case Study 5.2.1 Leveling up: Mass-media campaigns for prevention of NCDs

Mass-media campaigns can change risk behavior by providing information with messages of warning, empowerment, or support, or offering incentives intended to correct erroneous normative beliefs, clarify social and legal norms, or set positive role models or social norms.[11] Several behavioral theories explain the possible relationships through which mass-media interventions can influence health-related behavior by improving knowledge, attitudes and self-efficacy that contribute to a person's motivation and competence to take appropriate

10 K. M. Venkat Narayan et al., 'Diabetes: The Pandemic and Potential Solutions', in *Disease Control Priorities in Developing Countries, 2nd Edition* (Washington, DC: Oxford University Press, New York The International Bank for Reconstruction and Development/The World Bank, 2006).

11 Marica Ferri et al., 'Media Campaigns for the Prevention of Illicit Drug Use in Young People', *Cochrane Database of Systematic Reviews*, 5.6 (2013), CD009287, https://doi.org/10.1002/14651858.CD009287.pub2

actions.[12] Given their potential for population reach, many governments often use mass media to deliver health messages with the intention of improving health literacy and mitigating risky health behavior.

The WHO recommends several mass-media campaigns as Best Buys in NCD prevention.[13] These include:

- mass-media campaigns that educate the public about the harms of smoking/tobacco use and second-hand smoke;
- mass-media campaigns to promote healthy diets (including social marketing to reduce the intake of total fat, saturated fats, sugars and salt) and the intake of fruits and vegetables;
- reduced salt intake through a mass-media campaign that aims to change behavior; or
- a mass-media campaign combined with other community-based education, motivational and environmental programs aimed at supporting behavioral change in relation to physical activity levels.

But mass-media interventions might be Contestable Buys. These campaigns are often implemented at relatively high cost, especially when they are administered though newspapers or other printed materials, radio, television, billboards or social media. Our review of three Cochrane publications[14] reveals that the available evidence is inadequate to conclude that mass-media campaigns alone can

---

12 Jane T. Bertrand et al., 'Systematic Review of the Effectiveness of Mass Communication Programs to Change HIV/AIDS-Related Behaviors in Developing Countries', *Health Education Research*, 21.4 (2006), 567–97, https://doi.org/10.1093/her/cyl036; Jeff Niederdeppe et al., 'Media Campaigns to Promote Smoking Cessation among Socioeconomically Disadvantaged Populations: What Do We Know, What Do We Need to Learn, and What Should We Do Now?', *Social Science and Medicine*, 67 (2008), 1343–53, https://doi.org/10.1016/j.socscimed.2008.06.037

13 David E. Bloom et al., *From Burden to 'Best Buys': Reducing the Economic Impact of Non-Communicable Diseases in Low-and Middle-Income Countries* (Geneva, 2011), http://apps.who.int/medicinedocs/documents/s18804en/s18804en.pdf

14 Malgorzata M. Bala et al., 'Mass Media Interventions for Smoking Cessation in Adults', *Cochrane Database of Systematic Reviews*, 2013, https://doi.org/10.1002/14651858.CD004704.pub3; Malcolm P. Brinn et al., 'Mass Media Interventions for Preventing Smoking in Young People', in *Cochrane Database of Systematic Reviews*, ed. by Kristin V. Carson (Chichester, UK: John Wiley & Sons, Ltd, 2010), https://doi.org/10.1002/14651858.CD001006.pub2; Annhild Mosdøl et al., 'Targeted Mass Media Interventions Promoting Healthy Behaviours to Reduce Risk of Non-Communicable Diseases in Adult, Ethnic Minorities', *Cochrane Database*

meaningfully change health behavior and/or reduce the burden of NCDs in the target population. Most studies related to mass-media campaigns that are focused on knowledge, attitude, awareness and short-term change in other outcomes (such as service utilizations) lack clear evidence about improvements in health outcomes (such as a reduction in the incidence or prevalence of NCDs).[15] There is therefore a need for stringent evaluation of such mass-media campaigns, using studies with a before-and-after design that control for all factors affecting the campaign. They should include qualitative methods to demonstrate impact and unpack the most important elements of the campaigns.[16] Mass-media campaigns may have become an established intervention by now, so it could be difficult for NCD managers to accept their failure in terms of evidenced direct health impact. Campaigns may also, however, have value to NCD managers because they generate social and political coverage and may open avenues to engage public support for more effective NCD policies.

This case shows that while mass campaigns are not clear Wasted Buys, targeted mass-media campaigns on their own are inadequate to moderate the growth of NCDs. It is better for these campaigns to be implemented after careful research that supports their use rather than relying on well-meaning but essentially blind faith. This case study lies in Quadrant A (Fig. 5.1) in the area of uncertainty.

Case Study 5.2.2 Overseas and over here: Cost-effectiveness of medical primary prevention strategies to reduce the risk of cardiovascular disease (CVD) in Tanzania

Following the publication of the WHO's CVD preventive guidelines,[17] a research team led by Tanzania's Ministry of Health and Social Welfare

---

of Systematic Reviews, 12.2 (2017), 200 https://doi.org/10.1002/14651858.CD011683.pub2

15 Ruth G. Jepson et al., 'The Effectiveness of Interventions to Change Six Health Behaviours: A Review of Reviews', *BMC Public Health*, 10.1 2010, https://doi.org/10.1186/1471-2458-10-538

16 Melanie A. Wakefield, Barbara Loken and Robert C. Hornik, 'Use of Mass Media Campaigns to Change Health Behaviour', *The Lancet*, 376.9748 (2010), 1261–1271, https://doi.org/10.1016/S0140-6736(10)60809-4

17 World Health Organization, *Prevention of Cardiovascular Disease: Guidelines for Assessment and Management of Total Cardiovascular Risk*, Nonserial Publication (Geneva, Switzerland: World Health Organization, 2011).

conducted a study on the cost-effectiveness of medical preventive therapies for reducing the absolute risk of CVD.[18] Although global evidence reflecting the benefits of preventive medicine in cardiology exists, variation in countries' circumstances, including demographic, epidemiological, socio-economic and policy contexts, limits the transferability of findings. The Ministry therefore collaborated with academics to produce a local cost-effectiveness study using local data, age-specific background mortality rates and the provider cost of CVD treatment.

The study found that Losartan and Simvastatin, as a combination drug for all risk levels, was successful in averting DALYs. However, Tanzania's willingness to pay (at that time 610 USD or 1 GDP per capita per DALY averted) was insufficient to warrant proceeding. A recommendation followed that medical treatment should not be provided for low-risk patients without diabetes. This combination drug seemed to be a Wasted Buy. In this case, the threshold was a major determinant in the decision-making process and was explicitly used to identify Wasted Buys.

Tanzania's study result lies in Section 1 of Quadrant B (Fig. 5.1) because primary prevention intervention is effective but the costs exceed the threshold. This is an example of an intervention that is effective but not cost-effective. If policy-makers were to increase the level of health investment, this would imply higher thresholds and the multi-drug combination may then prove to be good value for money (however, doing this would also increase the likely cost-effectiveness of other, possibly even more efficient, interventions).

Case Study 5.2.3 Streamlining health policy for health gains: Diabetes screening in Thailand and Indonesia

A large element of the NCD burden in Southeast Asia is attributed to diabetes. An estimated 96 million people have diabetes, 90% of whom have the preventable type 2 diabetes.[19] Almost half this burden goes

18 Frida N. Ngalesoni et al., 'Cost-Effectiveness of Medical Primary Prevention Strategies to Reduce Absolute Risk of Cardiovascular Disease in Tanzania: A Markov Modelling Study', *BMC Health Services Research*, 16.1 (2016), 1–29, https://doi.org/10.1186/s12913-016-1409-3

19 'Addressing Asia's Fast Growing Diabetes Epidemic', *Bulletin of the World Health Organization*, 95.8 (2017), 550–51, https://doi.org/10.2471/blt.17.020817

undetected, especially among disadvantaged minorities. However, timely diagnosis eases diabetes management and ensures access to appropriate care. Several countries have implemented population-based diabetic screening programs. One such program is the WHO Package of Essential Non-communicable Disease Interventions (WHO PEN). The tools in this package enable early detection and management of the major NCDs. Although screening is widely considered to be an effective strategy, program managers and policy-makers often fail to assess the transferability of the global guidelines.

In Indonesia and Thailand, CVD and diabetes are significant disease burdens. Given the health and financial benefits of screening, these countries' ministries adapted parts of the PEN guidelines for their primary care public health services. After three years of implementation, an economic evaluation of the PEN package in Indonesia compared to no screening was conducted.[20] The findings revealed that implementation of the PEN program was indeed better than no policy, although it could have been improved through a targeted screening policy for high-risk groups aged forty and above, as opposed to the current entry level of fifteen years old. Screening for the fifteen-to-thirty-nine-year-old age category turned out to be a Wasted Buy. The savings from adopting the study recommendations could potentially be invested wisely and efficiently in other areas of priority.

In 2012, Thailand introduced a policy for national diabetes screening annually for people aged fifteen years and above. The policy was solely based on a high-level decision-maker's judgement following an analysis of the national epidemiological survey, but without considering other important factors such as infrastructure, feasibility, readiness assessment, or affordability. In 2015, an economic evaluation found that a targeted screening program for people aged thirty years and above would be more efficient.[21] Here again, screening the fifteen-to-thirty-year-old segment of the population was found to be a Wasted Buy.

---

20 Waranya Rattanavipapong et al., 'One Step Back, Two Steps Forward: An Economic Evaluation of the PEN Program in Indonesia', *Health Systems and Reform*, 2.1 (2016), 84–98, https://doi.org/10.1080/23288604.2015.1124168

21 Yot Teerawattananon et al., 'Development of a Health Screening Package under the Universal Health Coverage: The Role of Health Technology Assessment', *Health Economics (United Kingdom)*, 25 (2016), 162–78, https://doi.org/10.1002/hec.3301

The adoption of the new targeted screening policy in Thailand, despite its practicality and financial feasibility, posed a major challenge to policy-makers due to a potential negative public perception of the disinvestment. In Thailand, even though the evaluation was conducted in 2015, implementation took three years and received much resistance from policy-makers. In cases like these, an assessment of the key success factors, as well as the external factors influencing the intervention and their implications in the implementation context, should be considered. Using the SEED Tool detailed in Chapter 3, Considerations Two and Three would help address these points systematically.

Diabetes screening lies in the cost-ineffective region of Section 1 of Quadrant B (Fig. 5.1), because, although screening can be cost-effective, screening the entire population is not.[22]

Case Study 5.2.4 Back to basics: Drug testing in Bhutan

Lifestyle choices contribute greatly to the burden of NCDs. Smoking, substance and alcohol abuse are notorious culprits. Some countries use workplace drug testing as a common intervention to mitigate the risk of substance abuse. The United States, one of the early adopters, first implemented it in the mid-1980s to ensure drug-free federal workplaces, initially for employees in safety and security jobs. Soon after, new laws allowed public and private companies to drug test their employees.[23] Decades later, other countries, including the United Kingdom, Canada and several other European countries, introduced measures allowing drug testing using urine sampling. The reliability of this method is imperfect. Urine drug testing can involve samples that have been diluted; it is unable to differentiate between recreational and habitual use or uses on or without prescription. It is also found that urine samples contain metabolites and little of the parent drug.[24]

---

22 Rattanavipapong et al.; Teerawattananon et al.; Wangchuk Dukpa et al., 'Is Diabetes and Hypertension Screening Worthwhile in Resource-Limited Settings? An Economic Evaluation Based on a Pilot of a Package of Essential Non-Communicable Disease Interventions in Bhutan', *Health Policy and Planning*, 30.8 (2015), 1032–43, https://doi.org/10.1093/heapol/czu106

23 Michael R. Frone, *Alcohol and Illicit Drug Use in the Workforce and Workplace, Choice Reviews Online* (Washington, DC: American Psychological Association, 2013).

24 Michael R. Levine and W. P. Rennie, 'Pre-Employment Urine Drug Testing of Hospital Employees: Future Questions and Review of Current Literature', *Occupational and Environmental Medicine*, 61.4 (2004), 318–24, https://doi.org/10.1136/oem.2002.006163

There are often two main objectives in implementing a drug testing program: to reduce substance abuse in the workplace during working hours; or to ensure workplace safety. The effectiveness of workplace drug testing in meeting these objectives is unclear or may have unintended negative outcomes. Two systematic reviews examined the effectiveness of random drug testing aimed at determining whether it reduces injuries and accidents, of which one also examined whether it deterred employee drug use. The studies had methodological limitations and the evidence was insufficient to conclude that drug testing was effective.[25] Several studies also found weaknesses in the reviews, such as lack of randomization and test result validation. Drug testing as an intervention should therefore be undertaken with caution.[26] In the United States, research shows that employee drug testing often does not reduce employee substance abuse but may have the effect of excluding abusers from the workplace entirely.[27] If the goal is to reduce substance abuse by individual employees and ensure that they are on the path to quitting, additional measures are needed to provide guidance and therapy for current drug users, whose cost-effectiveness would also of course require testing. Screening alone appears to have little to no bearing on quitting rates.

These issues do not disappear when LMICs implement similar policies without thoroughly examining the evidence. Bhutan implemented a pre-employment drug-testing scheme for its Royal Civil Service

25 C. M. Cashman et al., 'Alcohol and Drug Screening of Occupational Drivers for Preventing Injury', *Cochrane Database of Systematic Reviews*, 2.13 (2009), https://doi.org/10.1002/14651858.cd006566.pub2; Timothy Christie, 'A Discussion of the Ethical Implications of Random Drug Testing in the Workplace', *Healthcare Management Forum*, 28.4 (2015), 172–74, https://doi.org/10.1177/0840470415581251; Michael T. French et al., 'To Test or Not to Test: Do Workplace Drug Testing Programs Discourage Employee Drug Use?', *Social Science Research Academic Press*, 2006, 33.1, 45–63, https://doi.org/10.1016/s0049-089x(03)00038-3

26 P. Homo et al., 'Workplace Drug Testing: An Overview of the Current Situation', *Journal of Toxins*, 3.1 (2016), https://doi.org/10.13188/2328-1723.1000013; Isabel Kazanga et al., 'Prevalence of Drug Abuse among Workers: Strengths and Pitfalls of the Recent Italian Workplace Drug Testing (WDT) Legislation', *Forensic Science International*, 215.1 (2012), 46–50, https://doi.org/10.1016/j.forsciint.2011.03.009; Hilde Marie Erøy Lund et al., 'Results of Workplace Drug Testing in Norway', *Norsk Epidemiologi*, 21.1 (2011), 55–59, https://doi.org/10.5324/nje.v21i1.1426; Michael T. French et al.; Shin Yu Lin et al., 'Urine Specimen Validity Test for Drug Abuse Testing in Workplace and Court Settings', *Journal of Food and Drug Analysis*, 26.1 (2018), 380–84, https://doi.org/10.1016/j.jfda.2017.01.001

27 Christie, 'A Discussion of the Ethical Implications of Random Drug Testing in the Workplace'.

Commission (RCSC).[28] The RCSC aimed to eliminate substance abuse in the government as well as to support the general national effort to deter abuse. The policy suffered some of the pitfalls mentioned above: 1) the tests were administered by human resource officers without adequate quality checks of the results; 2) while the twenty-four-hour notification to the employee prior to testing was a rule, the actual implementation was questionable; 3) of the 1,682 new employees in 2017, only two tested positive, so the positive test rate was low, which might be accurate or might be due to prevalent false negative test results; and 4) though the employees were sent to a Drugs Counselling Centre for guidance, there were no further measures. Further, there are no concrete interventions to address substance abuse by current employees.

The SEED Tool recommends that one should first examine the theoretical grounds for implementation as well as the existing evidence to ascertain the policy's a priori viability in meeting its aims. Given that there are clinical and implementation issues as well as weak evidence for this intervention, the NCD managers could choose to revise the policy or change it entirely. For example, other interventions, such as health promotion detailing the dangers of substance abuse and intensive therapy, could be implemented alongside the testing. This case lies in Quadrant A as a Wasted Buy near or in the area of uncertainty (Fig. 5.1).

5.3 Common Features of Wasted Buys

These case studies reveal common features of Wasted Buys. They often result from misguided motivations and beliefs, as well as from political, institutional, managerial, economic and social pressures and rigidities pervading the decision-making and implementation sphere of NCD management. The following summarizes some of the main features: 1) the fallacy that prevention interventions are always Best Buys; 2) one size seldom fits all in international guidelines; 3) policy-based evidence versus evidence-based policy; 4) selective implementation of interventions; and 5) low CE threshold used for decision-making.

28 RCSC, 'Notifcation-on-Drug-Test', 2017, https://www.rcsc.gov.bt/wp-content/uploads/2017/08/Notifcation-on-Drug-Test.pdf; RCSC, 'Bhutan Civil Service Rules and Regulations', 2018, https://www.rcsc.gov.bt/wp-content/uploads/2018/05/BCSR2018.pdf

5.3.1 The Fallacy that Prevention Interventions Are Always Best Buys

The case studies show that NCD managers, decision-makers and stakeholders are vulnerable to an inaccurate generalization to the effect that preventive interventions are always both effective and cost-effective and so can significantly reduce the burden of the disease (the 'prevention is better than cure' mantra). Such beliefs persist because of a lack of reliable evidence about the true impact of prevention. Many also believe that national scaling-up of a preventive intervention increases the benefits gained. This may not always be the case, as was found in Indonesia and Thailand's diabetic screening of a young population.

5.3.2 One Size Seldom Fits All in International Guidelines

It is evident from the case studies in Indonesia, Tanzania and Thailand, as well as from many other countries not described here, that there is much uncritical adoption of international recommendations and guidelines in the belief that they are a gold standard. Even when they develop their own guidelines, countries tend to incorporate international recommendations without contextualization. Disease factors and incidence, health-system infrastructure and the cost of intervention often change the calculated cost-effectiveness of interventions. Uncritical acceptance of studies done in other, more developed countries imparts a systematic bias when applying results to LMICs. This is a problem of the transferability of prevention guidelines from one setting to another. International recommendations are rarely tailored to the economic levels of countries, whether low-income, upper/middle-income, or high-income. They are generally based on an analysis of all countries with a natural focus around the mean. In this case, recommendations may be applicable to half of all countries that require them, but not to the rest (see Fig. 5.2) — for example, in the case of evaluating an anti-hypertensive medicine with a price range that varies globally. While this seems like a doom-and-gloom scenario for countries beginning the formulation of their NCD programs, international guidelines can still be a useful starting point for policy consideration and priority-setting — but they do require careful scrutiny of methods and evidence, and may sometimes require detailed analysis of subgroups via a systematic review or, whenever feasible, further locally-focused research.

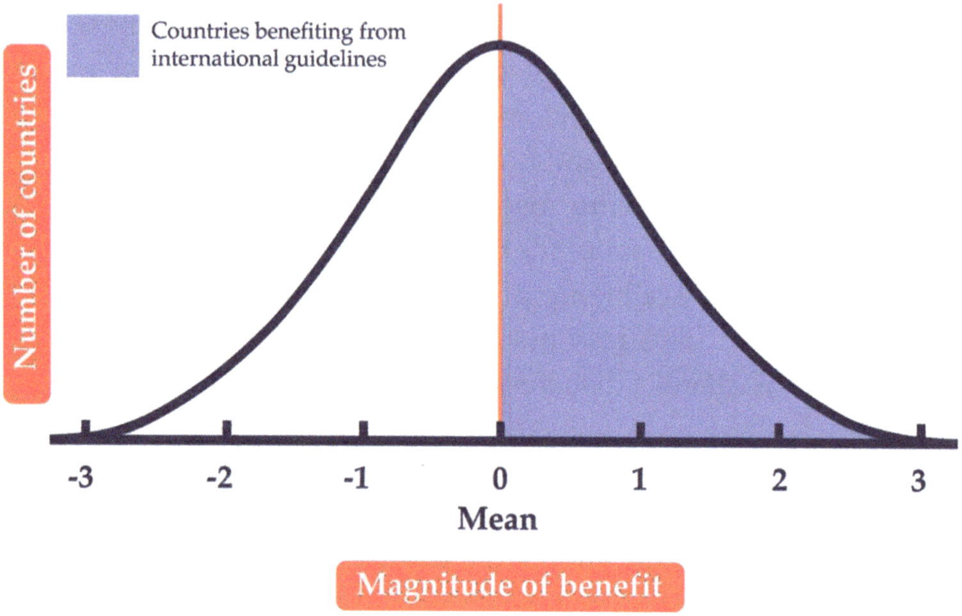

Fig. 5.2 Normal distribution of countries benefitting from international guidelines.

5.3.3 Policy-Based Evidence Versus Evidence-Based Policy

Policies can sometimes be developed without strong evidential support, because they are supported instead by the interests or passions of high-level decision-makers, or by pressures from stakeholder groups. Such policies are likely to result in Wasted Buys. For example, one case study demonstrated that a high-level politician was a zealous supporter of diabetes mellitus screening, for which they then sought evidence to support implementation. This selective use of evidence is a form of exclusion bias. While 'political engagement and support' is an extremely important part of the policy-making process and is required to implement the policy, the SEED Tool places it as a final check to prevent 'policy-based evidence' and reduce the likelihood of a Wasted Buy.

5.3.4 Selective Implementation of Interventions

NCDs are complex diseases requiring multi-layered interventions. However, some case studies, such as the Bhutan drug-testing program and the mass-media campaign for NCD prevention, make it evident that countries often implement an intervention, policy or technology that is untested or has conflicting or unconvincing evidence of effectiveness. This scenario may be due in part to the first common feature of Wasted Buys, which is a belief in preventive interventions as inevitable Best Buys. A related case is the implementation of interventions that have positive effects but have been shown to require additional interventions to ensure a more substantial impact relative to other interventions, or that are effective but too costly. 'Too costly' in this context means that a greater health benefit would have been generated had the money been spent on other interventions, or in other sectors. This is a classic area where an 'on-paper' Best Buy results in either a Contestable or Wasted Buy due to incomplete understanding of the cost-effectiveness criterion, pre-judgment and bias, inappropriate inferences about studies that have been done elsewhere and poor or incomplete implementation.

5.3.5 Low CE Threshold Used for Decision-Making

Even a threshold that is low by international standards of cost-effectiveness can cause an intervention to be a Wasted Buy because a threshold that is not set *sufficiently* low will lead to more recommended additions to the benefits package than the budget can sustain. There are many ways of determining this threshold.[29] The right threshold may be hard to discern but it should not be set arbitrarily. An ICER that admits more interventions than are affordable is too high, so the judgment of affordability (i.e., what the budget will support) is very important. It is much more common for thresholds, whether explicit or implicit, to be set too high than too low. One way of judging the right level of the threshold is to model the likely consequence of (a) small rises or falls in it and (b) small rises or falls in the healthcare budget allocation. Such experimentation ought to indicate clearly whether the threshold should be set higher or lower.[30] The tendency to set thresholds too high encourages Wasted Buys and may cause true Best Buys to be crowded out by interventions that have a much lower impact on the public's health.

29 See Chapter 1.

30 Anthony J. Culyer, 'Cost-Effectiveness Thresholds in Health Care: A Bookshelf Guide to Their Meaning and Use', *Health Economics, Policy and Law*, 11.4 (2016), 415–32, https://doi.org/10.1017/s1744133116000049

5.4 Recommendations

Our goal has been to assist NCD managers and other stakeholders in navigating a pathway from Wasted to Best Buys in their own local context. But what ought one to do to correct past commitments to Wasted Buys that are still present in the system? The science of 'reversing' such commitments is evolving, but the intellectual guidance provided in this Wasted-Buy chapter still holds. To avoid future Wasted Buys, or to reverse an existing one, requires similar analysis and a similar commitment. There needs to be:

- due deliberation about the additional[31] considerations;
- collective acknowledgment of the existence of Wasted Buys — that they may entail sunk costs but nevertheless are diverting resources from higher-value applications;
- an awareness that it is critical to generate good will — political, professional and social — for broader stakeholder support and the process of carrying out reform, involving ongoing stakeholder consultation and participation;
- a high-level commitment to ensure that priority-setting is part of an explicit, formal and well-resourced policy agenda beyond short-term political timelines;
- transparent decision-making frameworks removed from vested interests;
- clear objectives and nomenclature, articulating an ethic of waste reduction and minimizing opportunity costs rather than rationing;
- and finally, substantial new resources for data collection, monitoring, analysis and sharing.[32]

Further, and to conclude, we recommend the following principles when considering any intervention:

31 See Chapter 4.

32 Adam G. Elshaug et al., 'Levers for Addressing Medical Underuse and Overuse: Achieving High-Value Health Care', *The Lancet*, 390.10090 (2017), 191–202, https://doi.org/10.1016/s0140-6736(16)32586-7

- follow the step-by-step SEED Tool for considering whether to implement an intervention or not. Not all preventive measures, even those recommended in international guidelines, can be assumed to be Best Buys — their health impact (relative to other opportunities) may not be worth the investment, depending on a variety of contextual factors;
- develop agendas and policies in a participatory and systematic way with adequate checks and balances and involvement of all relevant stakeholders, to increase policy scrutiny and reduce the likelihood of 'policy-based evidence';
- consider whether the reason why an intervention might be cost-ineffective, and therefore a Wasted Buy, could be related to the cost and outcome components. For example, the intervention cost may be higher in the implementation setting compared to the study setting;
- seek ways of turning an intervention into a Best Buy, such as cutting or minimizing high-cost items without adversely affecting effectiveness. Identify the factors affecting outcomes and whether there are contextual circumstances that limit the impact of the intervention;
- consider whether there is a tenable case for a selective intervention even though, based on evidence, it should be coupled with other interventions as part of a package to address the outcome;
- lastly, if the intervention has a relatively low ICER but remains cost-ineffective according to the average thresholds used in the literature, consider whether the average threshold is even roughly appropriate for your setting.

6. Assessing the Transferability of Economic Evaluations
A Decision Framework

David D. Kim, Rachel L. Bacon and Peter J. Neumann

6.1 Introduction

As the field of economic evaluation has grown, questions have arisen about how 'transferable' or 'generalizable' studies are across settings. Part of the answer may lie in improving standards for economic evaluation. Various organizations and groups have proposed standard practices ('reference case analyses') to ensure transparency, high quality and comparability across cost-effectiveness analyses.[1] Over the past decade, many high-income countries have also developed their own standards and guidelines.[2] On the other hand, despite increasing use of

1 Tessa-Tan-Torres Edejer et al., 'Making Choices in Health: WHO Guide to Cost-Effectiveness Analysis', 2003, (Geneva: World Health Organization), https://www.who.int/choice/publications/p_2003_generalised_cea.pdf; Gillian D. Sanders et al., 'Recommendations for Conduct, Methodological Practices, and Reporting of Cost-Effectiveness Analyses: Second Panel on Cost-Effectiveness in Health and Medicine', *JAMA*, 316.10 (2016), 1093–103, https://doi.org/10.1001/jama.2016.12195; Thomas Wilkinson et al., 'The International Decision Support Initiative Reference Case for Economic Evaluation: An Aid to Thought', *Value Health*, 19.8 (2016), 921–28, https://doi.org/10.1016/j.jval.2016.04.015

2 Randa Eldessouki and Marilyn Dix Smith, 'Health Care System Information Sharing: A Step toward Better Health Globally', *Value in Health Regional Issues*, 1.1 (2012), 118–20, https://doi.org/10.1016/j.vhri.2012.03.022; Yot Teerawattananon, 'Thai Health Technology Assessment Guideline Development', *Journal of the Medical Association of Thailand*, 91.6 (2011), 11; Pharmaceutical Benefits Advisory Committee, *Guidelines for Preparing Submissions to the Pharmaceutical Benefits Advisory*

 https://doi.org/10.11647/OBP.0195.06

economic evaluations for priority-setting and reimbursement decisions,[3] local guidelines have only recently emerged among low- and middle-income countries (LMICs).[4] To fill the gap, the international Decision Support Initiative (iDSI), with the support of the Bill and Melinda Gates Foundation, has provided a 'reference case' for economic evaluations to reflect best practices and guidelines that could apply to different contexts, particularly in LMICs.[5]

Still, questions about transferability remain. In recent years, the number of available CEAs employing disability-adjusted life-years (DALYs) has grown rapidly (Fig. 6.1). These analyses typically reflect the context and health systems of a particular country or region. Ideally, local authorities in other areas, seeking to understand their own locally relevant Best or Wasted Buys and lacking an economic evaluation applied to their own jurisdictions, would conduct a new study to generate localized evidence. However, such authorities, particular in LMICs, often lack expertise and resources for producing such evidence.[6] As shown in Figure 6.2,[7] many LMICs have few or no economic studies available, thus highlighting the opportunity for decision-makers in these jurisdictions to apply economic evaluations conducted elsewhere.

Committee (PBAC) Version 5.0 (Canberra: Department of Health; 2016); Michael D. Rawlins and Anthony J. Culyer, 'National Institute for Clinical Excellence and Its Value Judgments', *BMJ: British Medical Journal*, 329.7459 (2004), 224–27, https://doi.org/10.1136/bmj.329.7459.224; Health Intervention and Technology Assessment Program (HITAP), *Guide to Health Economic Analysis and Research (GEAR) Online Resource: Guidelines Comparison*, 2019, http://www.gear4health.com/gear/health-economic-evaluation-guidelines

3 Catherine Pitt et al., 'Foreword: Health Economic Evaluations in Low- and Middle-Income Countries: Methodological Issues and Challenges for Priority Setting', *Health Econ*, 25 Suppl 1 (2016), 1–5, https://doi.org/10.1002/hec.3319

4 Health Intervention and Technology Assessment Program (HITAP); Benjarin Santatiwongchai et al., 'Methodological Variation in Economic Evaluations Conducted in Low-and Middle-Income Countries: Information for Reference Case Development', *PLoS One*, 10.5 (2015), e0123853, https://doi.org/10.1371/journal.pone.0123853

5 Wilkinson et al.

6 Michael F. Drummond et al., 'Issues in the Cross-National Assessment of Health Technology', *International Journal of Technology Assessment in Health Care*, 8.4 (1992), 670–82; M. Drummond, F. Augustovski et al., 'Challenges Faced in Transferring Economic Evaluations to Middle Income Countries', *International Journal of Technology Assessment in Health Care*, 31.6 (2015), 442–48, https://doi.org/10.1017/s0266462315000604

7 Center for the Evaluation of Value and Risk in Health (CEVR) Tufts Medical Center, Global Health CEA Registry, 2018, http://healtheconomics.tuftsmedicalcenter.org/ghcearegistry/

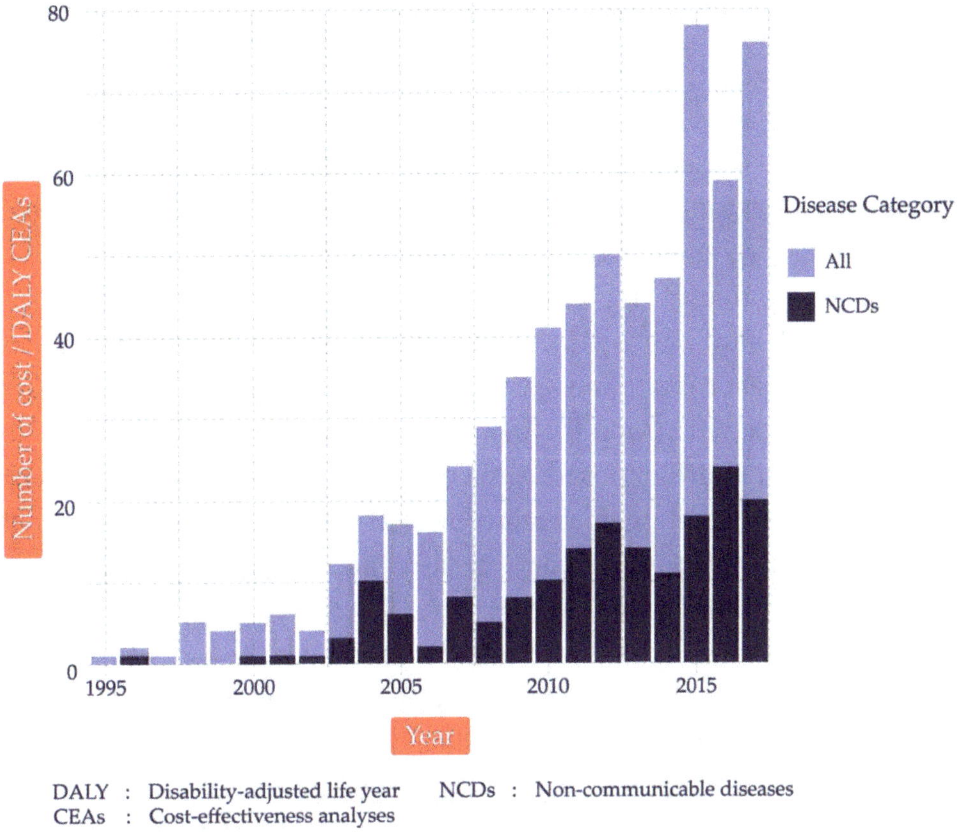

Fig. 6.1 The growth of cost-per-DALY-averted studies. Source: Author's analysis of Tufts Medical Center Global Health Cost-Effectiveness Analysis (CEA) Registry (www.ghcearegistry.org).

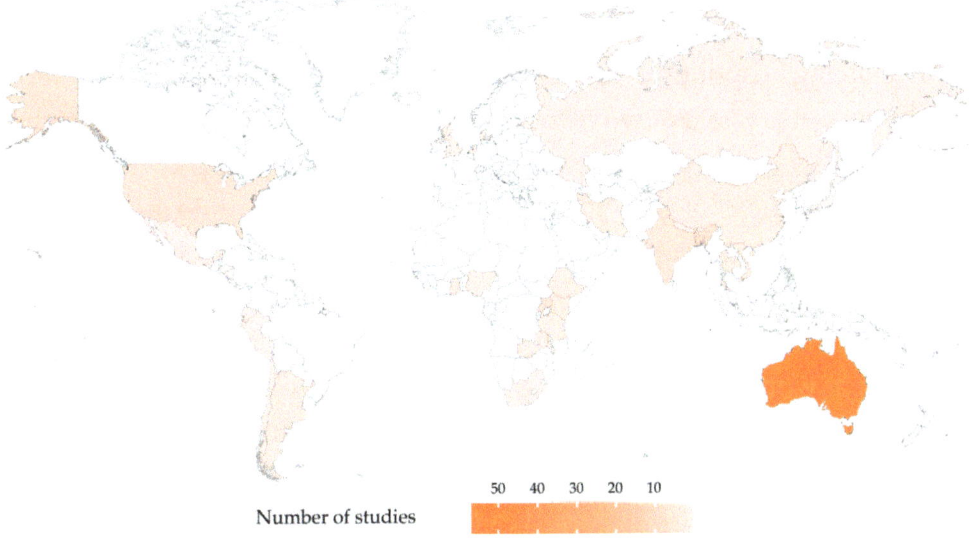

Fig. 6.2 Geographic distributions of available cost-per-DALY-averted studies for non-communicable diseases. Source: Author's analysis of Tufts Medical Center Global Health CEA Registry (www.ghcearegistry.org).

Note: DALY = disability-adjusted life-year.

When applying economic evidence generated elsewhere to local settings, researchers and decision-makers need to consider potentially important differences in factors such as population characteristics, epidemiology, relative prices, religion and culture, and health systems. For example, the economic value of implementing national breast cancer screening may vary substantially by the regional or local population risks of developing breast cancer; the feasibility of workplace health and safety measures will depend upon the work patterns that prevail and the risks to which workers are exposed; the costs and benefits associated with investing or disinvesting in fertility services or clinics for pregnancy terminations are likely to vary greatly according to predominant national religious affiliations.

For this chapter, we define 'transferability' as the extent to which particular study findings can be applied to another setting or context. Results from highly transferable studies could thus be used in various decision-making contexts without further adjustment.

Despite the importance of transferability in global health priority-setting, several major guidelines and reports, including the Disease Control Priorities Third Edition, do not explicitly address a process for evaluating transferability or list the factors to consider for local relevance.[8] This chapter provides a decision-making framework and a checklist for the field, to help local decision-makers and practitioners who wish to apply existing economic evaluation results to their own settings.

The chapter starts by reviewing the existing literature on the transferability of economic evaluations (Section 6.2). We then summarize critical factors for consideration and provide a decision-making framework to help determine whether local decision-makers should accept the external evidence without further adjustment, modify it to reflect local data, or reject it altogether (Section 6.3). Section 6.4 provides a worked example to provide a step-by-step illustration of how to perform the transferability assessment using our framework. We also discuss the use of an 'Impact Inventory' to aid decision-makers who wish to conduct for themselves original economic evaluations and identify Best and Wasted Buys in local settings (Section 6.5). The final section (Section 6.6) provides conclusions and future steps.

---

8 Wilkinson et al.; S. Horton, 'Cost-Effectiveness Analysis in Disease Control Priorities', in *Disease Control Priorities*, ed. by D. Jamison et al. (Washington, DC: World Bank, 2017), 3rd edn., IX, pp. 145–56.

6.2 Review of the Literature

A growing literature discusses issues surrounding the transferability of economic evaluations. Previous studies identified factors such as epidemiology, demography, relative prices, capacities of health systems, political and cultural conditions, affordability and others. These studies also suggested that the transferability of results to other settings was sometimes feasible, though a lack of transparency in the original research often made a judgment impossible. Several case studies have also been conducted to assess transferability empirically, for example, in physical activities among children, breast cancer treatment and smoking cessation.[9] Despite the substantial growth of studies on this topic, systematic literature reviews and national guidelines have highlighted variations in approaches regarding the transferability of data from one setting to another.[10] Here, we briefly summarize the contributions of major papers identified through Google Scholar, PubMed and cited references. Online Appendix 6A provides the search strategy in detail.

In 1992, Drummond and co-authors first highlighted important considerations for extrapolating economic evaluation results using a case study of a multi-country evaluation of the prophylactic use of misoprostol vs. no prophylaxis for patients with abdominal pain.[11] The paper suggested that a standard methodology used for all studies and

9 Saskia Knies et al., 'The Transferability of Economic Evaluations: Testing the Model of Welte', *Value Health*, 12.5 (2009), 730–38, https://doi.org/10.1111/j.1524-4733.2009.00525.x; Katharina Korber, 'Potential Transferability of Economic Evaluations of Programs Encouraging Physical Activity in Children and Adolescents across Different Countries — a Systematic Review of the Literature', *International Journal of Environmental Research and Public Health*, 11.10 (2014), 10606–21, https://doi.org/10.3390/ijerph111010606; Brigitte A. B. Essers et al., 'Transferability of Model-Based Economic Evaluations: The Case of Trastuzumab for the Adjuvant Treatment of HER2-Positive Early Breast Cancer in the Netherlands', *Value Health*, 13.4 (2010), 375–80, https://doi.org/10.1111/j.1524-4733.2009.00683.x; Marrit Berg et al., 'Model-Based Economic Evaluations in Smoking Cessation and Their Transferability to New Contexts: A Systematic Review', *Addiction*, 112.6 (2017), 946–67, https://doi.org/10.1111/add.13748

10 Ron Goeree et al., 'Transferability of Health Technology Assessments and Economic Evaluations: A Systematic Review of Approaches for Assessment and Application', *Clinicoeconomics and Outcomes Research*, 3 (2011), 89–104, https://doi.org/10.2147/CEOR.S14404; M. Angel Barbieri et al., 'What Do International Pharmacoeconomic Guidelines Say about Economic Data Transferability?', *Value Health*, 13.8 (2010), 1028–37, https://doi.org/10.1111/j.1524-4733.2010.00771.x

11 M. F. Drummond et al., *Issues in the Cross-National Assessment of Health Technology.*

the application of local data may facilitate the extrapolation process. In 1997, O'Brien summarized concerns about the transferability of cost-effectiveness data, underscoring six significant issues: demographics and the epidemiology of diseases; local clinical practice and conventions; incentives and regulations for providers; relative prices; patient preferences; and the opportunity costs of resources.[12]

Since the publication of these papers, several other investigators have suggested overarching frameworks, further explored key factors, and have begun to provide an empirical basis for understanding transferability. For example, Sculpher et al. systematically reviewed factors underlying variability in economic evaluations and recommended strategies for improving the generalizability of results.[13] Welte et al. developed a transferability decision chart that included 'knock-out' criteria and offered a transferability factor checklist as well as methods for improving transferability.[14] Boulenger et al. provided the European Network of Health Economics Evaluation Databases (EURONHEED) transferability information checklist.[15] Manca and Willan proposed algorithms to choose an appropriate methodology to address between-country differences.[16] Goeree et al. identified seventy-seven factors affecting transferability, which they grouped into five categories: the patient; the disease; the provider; the healthcare system; and methodological conventions.[17] In an attempt to improve the evaluation

12 Bernie J. O'Brien, 'A Tale of Two (or More) Cities: Geographic Transferability of Pharmacoeconomic Data', *Am J Manag Care*, 3 Suppl (1997), S33–9.

13 Mark J. Sculpher et al., 'Generalisability in Economic Evaluation Studies in Healthcare: A Review and Case Studies', *Health Technology Assessment*, 8.49 (2004), https://doi.org/10.3310/hta8490

14 Robert Welte et al., 'A Decision Chart for Assessing and Improving the Transferability of Economic Evaluation Results between Countries', *Pharmacoeconomics*, 22.13 (2004), 857–76, https://doi.org/10.2165/00019053-200422130-00004

15 Stephanie Boulenger et al., 'Can Economic Evaluations Be Made More Transferable?', *European Journal of Health Economics*, 6.4 (2005), 334–46, https://doi.org/10.1007/s10198-005-0322-1; John Nixon et al., 'Guidelines for Completing the EURONHEED Transferability Information Checklists', *European Journal of Health Economics*, 10.2 (2009), 157–65, https://doi.org/10.1007/s10198-008-0115-4

16 Andrea Manca and Andrew R. Willan, ''Lost in Translation': Accounting for Between-Country Differences in the Analysis of Multinational Cost-Effectiveness Data', *Pharmacoeconomics*, 24.11 (2006), 1101–19, https://doi.org/10.2165/00019053-200624110-00007

17 Ron Goeree et al., 'Transferability of Economic Evaluations: Approaches and Factors to Consider When Using Results from One Geographic Area for Another', *Current Medical Research Opinion*, 23.4 (2007), 671–82, https://doi.org/10.1185/030079906x167327

process, researchers have developed transferability indices to quantify the degree of transferability of economic evaluations.[18] An International Society for Pharmacoeconomics and Outcomes Research (ISPOR) Task Force Report reviewed national guidelines on transferability and made several recommendations for improvement.[19] A regional-specific assessment of transferability was conducted for middle-income countries,[20] Eastern Europe[21] and Latin America.[22]

Despite previous work to identify key factors and suggest frameworks for assessing transferability, existing tools may not be suited for local authorities due to the technical and complex nature of the assessment. Building upon past literature, we sought to develop a new decision framework and checklist for assessing the transferability of economic evidence to local settings (Section 6.3). Decision-makers and program managers often require rapid answers to complex questions. Our step-by-step guideline is a practical tool to compensate for the scarcity of locally-relevant economic evidence in many LMICs and to help assess the transferability of external evidence.

6.3 A Decision Framework for Identifying Locally-Relevant Best and Wasted Buys

6.3.1 Background

In Chapter 3, the authors describe a decision pyramid (the Systematic thinking for Evidence-based and Efficient Decision-making [SEED] Tool), which suggests exploring the transferability of economic

18 Boulenger et al.; Fernando Antonanzas et al., 'Transferability Indices for Health Economic Evaluations: Methods and Applications', *Health Economics*, 18.6 (2009), 629–43, https://doi.org/10.1002/hec.1397

19 Michael J. Drummond et al., 'Transferability of Economic Evaluations across Jurisdictions: ISPOR Good Research Practices Task Force Report', *Value in Health*, 12.4 (2009), 409–18, https://doi.org/10.1111/j.1524-4733.2008.00489.x

20 Michael Drummond et al., 'Challenges Faced in Transferring Economic Evaluations to Middle Income Countries', *International Journal of Technology Assessment in Health Care*, 31.6 (2015), 442–48, https://doi.org/10.1017/s0266462315000604

21 Olena Mandrik et al., 'Transferability of Economic Evaluations To Central and Eastern European and Former Soviet Countries', *Value in Health*, 17.7 (2014), A443-4, https://doi.org/10.1016/j.jval.2014.08.1172

22 G. Stewart et al., 'A Systematic Review of Economic Evaluations in Latin America: Assessing the Factors That Affect Adaptation and Transferability of Results', *Value in Health*, 18.7 (2015), A813, https://doi.org/10.1016/j.jval.2015.09.218

evidence (Consideration 3 of the SEED Tool) as part of a process for identifying Best and Wasted Buys. In this chapter, we provide a decision framework and assessment checklist to assess transferability objectively and transparently in a practical manner.

Before applying the framework and checklist, we recommend that evaluators, like NCD program managers, proceed only after identifying the following types of information: economic evaluations relevant for disease areas of interest (e.g., Best Buy interventions identified in Chapter 4); and local guidelines on economic evaluation to be used as a point of reference during assessment (if unavailable, we recommend international guidelines, such as the iDSI reference case).[23] Because assessments can be complex, we suggest convening a technical review panel that involves, if possible, a variety of stakeholders, such as epidemiologists, clinicians, disease program managers and analysts (e.g., decision scientists or modeling experts). A variety of expertise in the review panel can provide diverse perspectives on how best to determine the transferability of the evidence to the local context.

6.3.2 A Decision Framework and a Transferability Assessment Checklist

The process starts with an initial assessment to determine whether the existing study warrants further evaluation (Step 1), followed by a data transferability assessment (Step 2). Using the flowchart (Fig. 6.3), four options regarding transferability exist: 1) applying the external evidence without further adjustment; 2) modifying the economic evidence based on local data; 3) using the evidence with caution when the economic evidence is not necessarily highly transferable, but still deemed informative to the decision problem; and 4) rejecting the evidence altogether. Table 6.1 provides a transferability checklist tool. The case study (Section 6.4 in this chapter) illustrates how to apply our framework and conduct the transferability assessment by using the example of Best Buy interventions for diabetes prevention and management for Kenya.

23 Wilkinson et al.

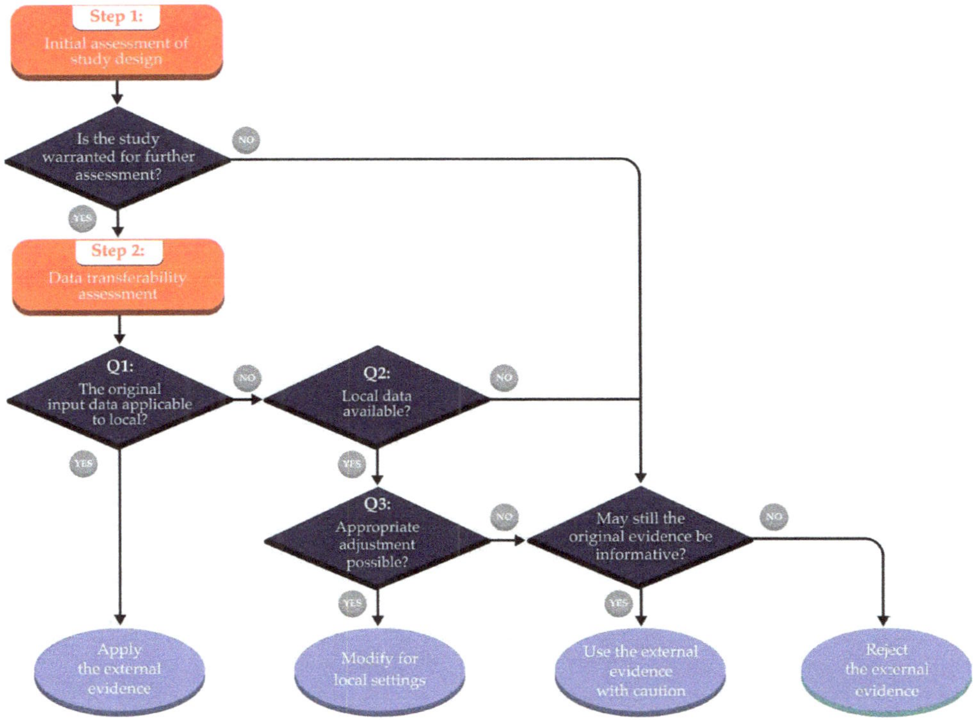

Fig. 6.3 Decision chart for assessing transferability and evidence review.

Table 6.1 Transferability assessment checklist.

Step 1: Initial assessment of study design			
Criteria	**Evaluation questions for each criterion**		**Decision Question:** Considering your evaluation for each criterion, is the original study warranted for the further assessment?
	Q1: Is the listed study characteristic aligned with local decision-making context? (If No, go to Q2)	Q2: Is the original study still informative to the decision problem?	
Study perspective			A. No, reject the external evidence
Intervention and its comparator(s)			B. No, but the external evidence can be used with caution
Time horizon			
Discounting			C. Yes, proceed to data transferability assessment (Step 2)
Study quality			

Step 2: Data transferability assessment					
Major considerations	**Evaluation questions for each data input**				**Decision Question:** Considering your evaluation for each criterion, is the original evidence transferable to your local setting?
	Q1: Are the original input data applied to the local setting? (If No, go to Q2)	Q2: Is local data on the specific input available? (If Yes, go to Q3 If No, go to Q4)	Q3: Is appropriate adjustment for local data input possible? (If No, go to Q4)	Q4: Is the data input used in the original study still informative to the local context?	
Baseline risk					A. No, reject the external evidence B. No, but the external evidence can be used with caution C. Yes, but only after appropriate adjustments for local data input D. Yes, apply the external evidence as it is
Treatment effects					
Unit costs/ prices					
Resource utilization					
Health-state preference weight					

Step 1: Initial Assessment of Study Design

A foundational starting point is to examine whether the study under consideration is a suitable candidate for the transferability assessment. Previous literature also describes this process as the minimal methodology standard or the set of 'knock-out' criteria.[24] The initial assessment consists of five components relevant to study design: A) perspective; B) intervention and its comparator(s); C) time horizon; D) discounting; and E) study quality. If any of these components do not meet the minimum criteria — which are subject to the evaluator's judgment — the study conclusion cannot be applied to local settings. However, when the original study results are judged as potentially useful (e.g., through sensitivity analyses reporting how Incremental Cost-Effectiveness Ratios [ICERs] vary by different perspectives), the evaluator may either apply the original findings with caution or proceed further to the data transferability assessment. We discuss each of the five components for minimum study standards in detail:

A. Study Perspective

Practice guidelines for economic evaluation emphasize the importance of the analytic perspective (or viewpoint) because it determines which costs and benefits to include in the analysis.[25] Analytic perspectives may reflect a specific payer (e.g., Ministry of Health or local government), the healthcare sector as a whole, or the broader society. Depending on the choice of perspective, an intervention may be more cost-effective (i.e., have a lower ICER) or less cost-effective. For example, pharmacotherapy for patients with alcohol use disorder is more cost-effective from a societal perspective than a healthcare sector perspective

24 Welte et al.; D. K. Heyland et al., 'Economic Evaluations in the Critical Care Literature: Do They Help Us Improve the Efficiency of Our Unit?', *Critical Care Medicine*, 24.9 (1996), 1591–98; Helmut Spath et al., 'Analysis of the Eligibility of Published Economic Evaluations for Transfer to a Given Health Care System. Methodological Approach and Application to the French Health Care System', *Health Policy*, 49.3 (1999), 161–77.

25 Michael F. Drummond et al., *Methods for the Economic Evaluation of Health Care Programmes* (Oxford: Oxford University Press, 2015); Peter J. Neumann et al., *Cost-Effectiveness in Health and Medicine* (New York: Oxford University Press, 2017).

because of improved outcomes that go beyond the healthcare sector, such as improved productivity or reduced alcohol-related motor-vehicle accidents.[26] We recommend that evaluators assess whether the study perspective aligns with their own decision-making preferences in their local setting.

B. Intervention and its Comparator(s)

Economic evaluation should reflect the specific decision problem that each individual decision-making group faces (e.g., interventions in routine use in the local setting). As a summary measure, the ICER represents the relative value between an intervention, which might already be available or considered for introduction in the local setting, and a comparator, which could be the standard of care, a comparable intervention, or the absence of an intervention. If the intervention or comparator(s) in the original study are not available or are not relevant in the local settings, results may not be easily transferable. Inadequate description of the intervention and comparator(s) in the original study may also limit transferability.

C. Time Horizon

The time horizon used in CEAs can substantially affect the estimated value of an intervention.[27] Standard guidelines recommend using a time horizon long enough to capture all relevant costs and health benefits.[28] When assessing interventions targeted for NCDs, such as cardiovascular diseases, cancer and diabetes, a lifetime horizon is recommended. Lifetime horizons can capture all of the important differences in consequences over time. For example, evaluators who wish to understand the economic

26 David D. Kim et al., 'Worked Example 1: The Costeffectiveness of Treatment for Individuals with Alcohol Use Disorders: A Reference Case Analysis', in *Cost-Effectiveness in Health and Medicine*, ed. by Peter J. Neumann et al. (New York: Oxford University Press, 2017), pp. 385–430.

27 David D Kim et al., 'The Influence of Time Horizon on Results of Cost-Effectiveness Analyses', *Expert Review of Pharmacoeconomics Outcomes Research*, 17.6 (2017), 615–23, https://doi.org/10.1080/14737167.2017.1331432.

28 Wilkinson et al.; Michael F Drummond et al., *Methods for the economic evaluation of health care programmes;* Neumann et al.

evidence on cardiovascular disease prevention may want to exclude studies conducted from a short-term horizon.

D. Discounting

Practice guidelines recommend discounting all future costs and health outcomes so that ICERs represent the 'present value' of the intervention, adjusting for the differential timing of costs and benefits.[29] In other words, discounting makes near-term consequences (e.g., immediate costs and health benefits) more valuable than long-term consequences (e.g., costs and health benefits occurring in distant future). This is because of the opportunity costs to spend money now and to experience immediate benefits instead of those in the future. The use of higher discounting rates (i.e., strongly devaluing distant costs and benefits) tends to underestimate the value of preventive interventions.

A discount rate reflects society's (or a specific decision-maker's) time preference (i.e., how much they are willing to trade off consumption today vs. tomorrow). Thus, guidelines sometimes suggest using the real rates of government bonds as a proxy. Despite the common use of 3% or 3.5% for discounting both costs and health outcomes (per guideline recommendations, such as iDSI reference case, designed to promote comparability across studies),[30] local evaluators may wish to select a time preference suitable for their country or context, or there may be standard rules set for all public-sector investment decisions.

E. Study Quality

When considering transferability, evaluators may understandably wish to exclude economic evaluations of low quality. The question is how to determine quality. Despite various guidelines and checklists on conducting and reporting CEAs,[31] challenges remain because these

29 Michael F. Drummond et al., *Methods for the economic evaluation of health care programmes*; Neumann et al.

30 Wilkinson et al.

31 Wilkinson et al.; Michael F. Drummond et al., *Methods for the Economic Evaluation of Health Care Programmes*; Sanders et al.; Don Husereau et al., 'Consolidated Health Economic Evaluation Reporting Standards (CHEERS) Statement', *BMJ*, 346 (2013), f1049, https://doi.org/10.1186/1741-7015-11-80; M. F. Drummond and T. O.

instruments are not designed to guide decision-makers on how to differentiate high- and low-quality studies. The quality of the study can be assessed based on adherence to the economic evaluation guidelines (the iDSI reference case or the Second Panel's recommendations) or via a formal quality assessment tool.[32] One source for such information is the Tufts Medical Center Global Health CEA Registry (www.ghcearegistry.org), which includes detail on the degree to which published cost-per-DALY-averted studies adhere to the iDSI reference case.[33]

Step 2: Data Transferability Assessment

After an initial screening, evaluators can determine, depending on data availability, whether the original evidence can be directly applied to their local setting. Despite a long list of items to be considered for data transferability, we focus on five major factors most often referred to in the literature: baseline risk, treatment effects, unit costs/prices, resource utilization and health-state preference weight. We will also briefly describe the other possible items for consideration.[34]

During the data assessment for each of the five factors, the evaluator will determine whether or not to progress to the next stage by doing a separate analysis in three key aspects. These aspects are: 1) the need for further adjustment; 2) the availability of local data; and 3) the possibility of adjustment based on information from the original study (e.g., in sensitivity analysis) or access to the original model (or authors) for further modification. In certain instances, evaluators may determine

---

Jefferson, 'Guidelines for Authors and Peer Reviewers of Economic Submissions to the BMJ. The BMJ Economic Evaluation Working Party', *BMJ*, 313.7052 (1996), 275–83; Alan Williams, 'The Cost-Benefit Approach', *Br Med Bull*, 30.3 (1974), 252–56; Zoë Philips et al., 'Good Practice Guidelines for Decision-Analytic Modelling in Health Technology Assessment: A Review and Consolidation of Quality Assessment', *Pharmacoeconomics*, 24.4 (2006), 355–71, https://doi.org/10.2165/00019053-200624040-00006

32 Sanders et al.; Wilkinson et al.; Joshua J. Ofman et al., 'Examining the Value and Quality of Health Economic Analyses: Implications of Utilizing the QHES', *J Manag Care Pharm*, 9.1 (2003), 53–61, https://doi.org/10.18553/jmcp.2003.9.1.53

33 Center for the Evaluation of Value and Risk in Health (CEVR) Tufts Medical Center; Joanna Emerson et al., 'Adherence to the IDSI Reference Case among Published Cost-per-DALY Averted Studies', *PLOS ONE*, 14.5 (2019), e0205633, https://doi.org/10.1371/journal.pone.0205633

34 Barbieri et al.; O'Brien; Sculpher et al.; Welte et al.; Boulenger et al.; Goeree et al.

that the original study is still informative to the local context even when the local data are not available or appropriate adjustment is not possible.

A. Baseline Risk (Disease Profile)

Variation in underlying population risk factors across countries is linked to different inherent baseline risk characteristics, such as differences in disease incidence, prevalence and background mortality. Differences in baseline risk may influence both an intervention's effects and its costs in terms of actual resource utilization. For example, implementing a nation-wide screening program for type 2 diabetes may generate more favorable ICERs for countries with a higher prevalence of undiagnosed type 2 diabetes.[35] Thus, the evaluator must determine whether the baseline risk in the original study is relevant to the local context.

B. Treatment Effects (Clinical Information)

Treatment effects (i.e., measured as an intervention's relative efficacy) are generally considered more transferable than other data inputs as the estimate is less likely to depend upon the practices and competencies of local professionals in LMICs and the incentive embodied in the local health system.[36] An estimate of the absolute treatment effect from a multinational, randomized controlled trial would presumably have high transferability. An estimate of the relative treatment effect may also be used from country-specific studies after an appropriate adjustment in local baseline risk.

C. Unit Costs/Prices

Adjusting for unit costs or prices relevant to the local context will typically be required for data transferability. Because of its importance,[37]

35 Thomas J. Hoerger et al., 'Screening for Type 2 Diabetes Mellitus: A Cost-Effectiveness Analysis', *Annals of International Medicine*, 140.9 (2004), 689–99, https://doi.org/10.7326/0003-4819-140-9-200405040-00008

36 Barbieri et al.

37 Barbieri et al.; Sculpher et al.; Welte et al.

economic evaluations often conduct sensitivity analyses on the prices of the intervention/comparator(s) as well as the prices for other services. Assuming that all other data inputs are relevant to the local setting, if the original study provides results from sensitivity analyses for a range of intervention prices, evaluators could extract the ICERs relevant to their local settings without re-analyzing the data. For example, when the price of a drug is $100 in the local setting, instead of $500 in the original study, an ICER from a sensitivity analysis (e.g., $1000/quality-adjusted life-years [QALY] gained at the drug price of $100) can be used as the locally relevant evidence, rather than the original evidence (e.g., $5000/QALY at the drug price of $500).

D. Resource Utilization

Similar to the case for unit costs, the application of locally-relevant resource use data (e.g., on hospital days, physician office visits, or medications) may be required for the estimation of overall costs associated with the intervention and comparator(s). Many international guidelines consider resource use data from external locations as inappropriate sources and strongly encourage the use of locally-relevant resource data.[38]

E. Health-State Preference Weight

Health-state preference weights, used as inputs into calculations of QALYs, represent the relative desirability for being in different health states. Guidelines generally recommend using generic preference measures (e.g., EQ-5D, SF-6D, or HUI) that assign a specific value to each health state, including zero for dead and one for perfect health.[39] Because of social and cultural factors, individuals in different countries

38 Barbieri et al.; Sculpher et al.; Boulenger et al.; Goeree et al.; Michael Drummond et al., 'Increasing the Generalizability of Economic Evaluations: Recommendations for the Design, Analysis, and Reporting of Studies', *International Journal of Technology Assessment in Health Care*, 21.2 (2005), 165–71, https://doi.org/10.1017/s0266462305050221

39 Michael F. Drummond et al., *Methods for the economic evaluation of health care programmes*; Neumann et al.

may assign different values to similar health states.[40] Previous studies have demonstrated that the valuations of health states can be different for US and UK residents and, as a result, cost-effectiveness ratios were doubled when adjusted to US-specific weights.[41]

For health-related quality of life measures used to calculate QALYs, thirty-two country-specific preference weights for EQ-5D (valuation sets) are currently available and the number continues to grow.[42] Disability weights, which are used to calculate DALYs, have been estimated from international survey participants. Although they may not reflect the preference for health states among specific target populations, disability weights may be more readily transferable across different countries.[43]

Once the data transferability assessment is completed, a final decision is required on whether local decision-makers should: 1) apply the external evidence without further adjustment, 2) modify the evidence based on local data, 3) use the evidence with caution because it is not highly transferable, but still deemed informative, or 4) reject the evidence altogether. In addition to the five major factors listed above, previous literature has described additional factors that may be relevant for assessing transferability.[44] The list includes variation in local clinical practice, healthcare infrastructure, cultural background, implementation costs and the valuation of productivity and other non-health benefits. When appropriate, evaluators may include additional factors for their data transferability assessments.

---

40 Francis Guillemin et al., 'Cross-Cultural Adaptation of Health-Related Quality of Life Measures: Literature Review and Proposed Guidelines', *Journal of Clinical Epidemiology*, 46.12 (1993), 1417–32, https://doi.org/10.1016/0895-4356(93)90142-n; Roger T. Anderson et al., 'A Review of the Progress towards Developing Health-Related Quality-of-Life Instruments for International Clinical Studies and Outcomes Research', *Pharmacoeconomics*, 10.4 (1996), 336–55, https://doi.org/10.2165/00019053-199610040-00004

41 Jeffrey A. Johnson et al., 'Valuations of EQ-5D Health States: Are the United States and United Kingdom Different?', *Medical Care*, 43.3 (2005), 221–28, https://doi.org/10.1097/00005650-200503000-00004; Katia Noyes et al., 'The Implications of Using US-Specific EQ-5D Preference Weights for Cost-Effectiveness Evaluation', *Medical Decision Making*, 27.3 (2007), 327–34, https://doi.org/10.1177/0272989X07301822

42 'EQ-5D Instruments — EQ-5D', https://euroqol.org/eq-5d-instruments/

43 Joshua A. Salomon et al., 'Disability Weights for the Global Burden of Disease 2013 Study', *Lancet Glob Health*, 3.11 (2015), e712–23, https://doi.org/10.1016/S2214-109X(15)00069-8

44 Sculpher et al.; Welte et al.

6.4 Worked Example: Assessing Transferability of Best Buy Interventions for Diabetes Prevention and Management in Kenya

6.4.1 Background and Rationale

To provide a step-by-step illustration of how to perform a transferability assessment using our framework and checklist, we offer a worked example from Kenya. We evaluated the transferability of seven studies for diabetes prevention and management,[45] which included fourteen interventions deemed Best Buys based on the WHO definition (i.e., cost-saving or ICER ≤ $100 international dollars (I$)/DALY averted). These interventions mostly include screening or interventions targeting behavioral changes (Table 6.2).

This worked example should be viewed as a stylized application, in order to provide an illustrative case study, rather than a definitive analysis for Kenya. Thus, throughout the example, we assume the role of a program manager for a hypothetical national diabetes prevention and control program in Kenya. The primary responsibility of the manager is to determine whether the identified Best Buy interventions for

45 Shukri F. Mohamed et al., 'Prevalence and Factors Associated with Pre-Diabetes and Diabetes Mellitus in Kenya: Results from a National Survey', *BMC Public Health*, 18.Suppl 3 (2018), 1215, https://doi.org/10.1186/s12889-018-6053-x; Sanjay Basu et al., 'Comparative Effectiveness and Cost-Effectiveness of Treat-to-Target versus Benefit-Based Tailored Treatment of Type 2 Diabetes in Low-Income and Middle-Income Countries: A Modelling Analysis', *Lancet Diabetes & Endocrinology*, 4.11 (2016), 922–32, https://doi.org/10.1016/s2213-8587(16)30270-4; Elliot Marseille et al., 'The Cost-Effectiveness of Gestational Diabetes Screening Including Prevention of Type 2 Diabetes: Application of a New Model in India and Israel', *Journal of Maternal-Fetal & Neonatal Medicine*, 26.8 (2013), 802–10, https://doi.org/10.3109/14767058.2013.765845; N. Lohse et al., 'Development of a Model to Assess the Cost-Effectiveness of Gestational Diabetes Mellitus Screening and Lifestyle Change for the Prevention of Type 2 Diabetes Mellitus', *International Journal of Gynaecology & Obstetrics*, 115 Suppl (2011), S20–5, https://doi.org/10.1016/s0020-7292(11)60007-6; Melanie Y. Bertram et al., 'Assessing the Cost-Effectiveness of Drug and Lifestyle Intervention Following Opportunistic Screening for Pre-Diabetes in Primary Care', *Diabetologia*, 53.5 (2010), 875–81, https://doi.org/10.1007/s00125-010-1661-8; Stephen Colagiuri and Agnes E. Walker, 'Using an Economic Model of Diabetes to Evaluate Prevention and Care Strategies in Australia', *Health Affairs (Millwood)*, 27.1 (2008), 256–68, https://doi.org/10.1377/hlthaff.27.1.256; Dana Goldman et al., 'The Value of Elderly Disease Prevention', *Forum Health Economics Policy*, 9.2 (2006), https://doi.org/10.2202/1558-9544.1004

diabetes prevention and management can be transferrable to Kenya and recommended as part of the country's essential health benefits package.

We selected Kenya as the target country for two reasons: 1) Kenya's recent move to Universal Health Coverage (UHC);[46] and 2) the rising burden of diabetes in the country.[47] Kenya's efforts to reform its health and finance system to achieve UHC have been the subject of media coverage.[48] However, barriers remain to achieving UHC in Kenya, specifically for NCD coverage, as infectious disease remains the focus of the government's funding and coverage expansions.[49] The burden of NCDs in Kenya has been rapidly increasing, accounting for 13,200 DALYs [36% of the country's overall disease burden in 2017, up from 25% in 1990). The prevalence of diabetes in Kenya was 2.4% in 2015,[50] and its burden is growing, accounting for 1.7% of total DALYs in 2017, up from 0.83% in 1990.[51]

6.4.2 Evaluator's Guideline on Economic Evaluation

To our knowledge, Kenya does not have local guidelines for conducting economic evaluations. For this stylized example, we selected the iDSI reference case as our hypothetical economic evaluation guideline for Kenya for the purpose of the transferability assessment.[52] Again, we note that the assumptions should be considered as illustrative and may not reflect actual context or preferences in Kenya.

---

46 Jemimah W. Mwakisha and O. K. A. Sakuya, *Building Health: Kenya's Move to Universal Health Coverage* (WHO Africa, 2018), https://www.afro.who.int/news/building-health-kenyas-move-universal-health-coverage

47 Global Burden of Disease Collaborative Network, *Global Burden of Disease Study 2017* (Seattle, United States: Institute for Health Metrics and Evaluation (IHME), 2019), http://ghdx.healthdata.org/gbd-results-tool

48 Jemimah W. Mwakisha and O. K. A. Sakuya; 'Focus on Infrastructure, Staffing as Kenya Rolls out Universal Healthcare', *Business Daily*, 2018, https://www.businessdailyafrica.com/datahub/Kenya-rolls-out-universal-healthcare/3815418-4889486-6tmjej/index.html; Elizabeth Merab, 'Road to UHC: What It Will Take to Achieve Health for All', *Daily Nation* (Nairobi City, Kenya, 2018), https://www.nation.co.ke/health/Road-to-UHC-what-it-will-take--to-achieve-health-for-all/3476990-4655230-jtp203z/index.html

49 Fredrick Nzwili, 'Kenya To Launch Universal Health Coverage Pilot Of Free Healthcare,' (Health Policy Watch, 2018), https://www.healthpolicy-watch.org/kenya-to-launch-universal-health-coverage-pilot-of-free-healthcare/

50 Mohamed et al.

51 Global Burden of Disease Collaborative Network.

52 Wilkinson et al.

For the initial assessment of study design (Step 1), our baseline decision making criteria were the following: 1) Study perspective: a societal perspective preferred, but healthcare payer (or government) perspective is acceptable; 2) Intervention and its comparator(s): the intervention under consideration should be available in the local setting; 3) Time horizon: a lifetime horizon is strongly preferred, but results from a shorter time horizon may also be considered with caveats; 4) Discounting: a 3% annual discount rate for both costs and health outcomes is preferred but results using different discounting rates may also be considered with a caveat; and 5) Study quality: poor study quality, which can be assessed based on adherence to the iDSI reference case guidelines,[53] is a reason for excluding a study from further assessment.

For the data transferability assessment (Step 2), considering our hypothetical role of a program manager for a national diabetes prevention and control program in Kenya, we assume that local data on baseline risk (i.e., disease profiles), unit costs/prices and resource utilization are readily available. Data on treatment effects or other relevant clinical information (e.g., diabetes risk prediction) are assumed to be transferable to Kenya in the absence of locally-relevant clinical data. Finally, we assume that use of disability weights, or health-related quality of life weights measured from local participants and valued using a local valuation set, is preferred, but measures or valuation sets from elsewhere can be used with a caveat. A summary of the hypothetical economic evaluation guideline for Kenya, on which our assessment is based, is available in the Online Appendix 6B.

6.4.3 Transferability Assessment Process

We conducted a transferability assessment as follows. Three evaluators on our research team with experience in cost-effectiveness analysis (a senior investigator and two junior researchers) formed our 'evaluation committee' to simulate the kind of transferability assessment that might occur in Kenya. The evaluation consisted of first reviewing: 1) the decision chart for assessing transferability (Fig. 6.3); 2) the transferability assessment checklist (Table 6.1); and 3) the hypothetical economic

53 Ibid.

Table 6.2 Assessing transferability of Best Buy interventions for diabetes prevention and management.

Study	Year	Intervention	Comparator	Study countries	Recommendations for transferability of external evidence to Kenya settings (Consensus statement)
Goldman	2006	Diabetes control (stated as: 'prevention,' and 'better treatment')	None	United States	The study finding is not transferable due to the failure to meet the minimum criteria for the study design evaluation. (e.g., no specific intervention was evaluated, no discounting rate was stated and low-quality score)
Colagiuri	2008	Screening for undiagnosed diabetes or pre-diabetes	None	Australia	Due to differences in key data inputs and the inability to adjust the original findings, the study finding is not directly transferable. However, the external evidence may be used with caution when reflecting local-level data (e.g., utilization rates).
Bertram	2010	Multiple interventions, 6 total: (1) pre-diabetes screening and diet and exercise; (2) pre-diabetes screening and exercise; (3) pre-diabetes screening and diet; (4) pre-diabetes screening and Acarbose; (5) pre-diabetes screening and Metformin; (6) pre-diabetes screening and Orlistat	Standard/usual care	Australia	Due to differences in key input data (e.g., Australian-specific disability weights were used), the study finding is not directly transferable. However, the external evidence may be used to (A) inform future research on the original cost-effectiveness study, or (B) pilot on a small scale to test for feasibility.

Lohse	2011	Gestational diabetes mellitus screening and lifestyle change	None	India; Israel	Given limited data on gestational diabetes and antenatal resource utilization, the study finding is not directly transferable. However, the study findings of cost-savings or favourable cost-effectiveness, which are applicable to a wide range of input values in India and Israel, may be used to inform resource allocation decisions in Kenya with caution. (India has a similar GDP per capita as Kenya)
Salomon	2012	Multiple interventions, 4 total: (1) lipid control; (2) blood pressure control; (3) conventional glycemic control; and (4) intensive glycemic control	None	Mexico	Reviewers both agreed that this is a high-quality study with great detail provided for key data inputs. With acknowledging that the study is based on the Mexican setting, the study findings could be used in Kenya settings after making reasonable substitutions based on local data, such as local prices.
Marseille	2013	Gestational diabetes mellitus screening using oral glucose tolerance test	None	India; Israel	Same recommendations as we made for Lohse et al., 2011. This study is an update of the existing study and reported similar results.
Basu	2016	Benefit-based tailored treatment (BTT) (which is based on a composite risk score of cardiovascular diseases or microvascular disease)	treat-to-target (TTT) strategy, which is based on achieving target levels of specific biomarkers (e.g., cholesterol level)	China; Ghana; India; Mexico; South Africa	Considering similarities between one of the study countries, Ghana and Kenya in terms of disease prevalence and economic profile, the external evidence is highly transferable and can be applied to inform resource allocation decisions in Kenya settings.

evaluation guideline for Kenya (Online Appendix 6B). After an initial training session, each of the three committee members independently conducted a transferability assessment for one of the seven articles[54] and then convened to review and discuss questions or challenges that arose during the assessment.

Once the two junior evaluators completed the basic training, they were 'commissioned' to evaluate the transferability of the remaining six articles independently. Next, they convened a consensus meeting to discuss whether the original study warranted further data assessment and, if so, whether the original evidence could be transferable to Kenya. Although each of the evaluators was encouraged to assess specific questions pertaining to the individual study characteristics and data inputs listed in Table 6.1, the final decision corresponded to one of four options: 1) apply the external evidence without further adjustment; 2) modify the evidence based on local data; 3) use the evidence with caution because the economic evidence was not necessarily highly transferable; and 4) reject the evidence altogether. During the consensus meeting, each of the members shared their individual decision and comments and the group discussed conflicting opinions to reach a consensus. Finally, the group made consensus recommendations for the transferability of the external evidence.

6.4.4 Transferability Assessment Results

Among seven studies evaluated, only one was deemed directly transferable to Kenya. In that case, the country of the original study, Ghana, was deemed sufficiently similar to Kenya in terms of disease prevalence and its economic profile.[55] The study found that a benefit-based tailored treatment, a strategy to reduce the composite risk of developing CVD in the next ten years or a microvascular disease risk over a lifetime for patients with type 2 diabetes, was a cost-saving strategy (i.e., lower costs with greater health benefits), compared to a treat-to-target strategy, which aimed to achieve target levels of specific biomarkers.

Our committee also decided that another study was not transferable due to its failure to meet the minimum criteria for the study design

54 Basu et al.

55 Ibid.

evaluation.[56] For example, although the original study reported that effective control of hypertension could avoid 75 million DALYs and reduce healthcare spending by $890 billion, the study did not examine any specific intervention to achieve effective hypertension control. The study's low-quality score (it neither stated its discount rate nor listed a specific intervention to be targeted) contributed to the committee's decision to reject the use of this evidence for Kenya.

For most of the other cases, study findings were deemed not directly transferable due to differences in key data inputs and an inability to adjust the original findings. However, the committee believed that the external evidence may still provide useful insight for how resources for diabetes prevention and management might best be allocated for Kenya, though caveats and caution were in order.

The initial assessment of the study design (Step 1) reached consensus with no disagreement. However, evaluation committee members were often unsure about the data transferability assessment (Step 2). Some of the assessment questions required knowledge about the availability of local data inputs and the accessibility of the models, which was not readily grasped by the committee members. During the consensus meeting, the evaluation committee resolved conflicts and ambiguity based on our guideline of transferability assessment designed for Kenya (the Online Appendix 6B). Table 6.2 provides our committee's consensus recommendations for the seven studies. The Online Appendix 6C provides the individual transferability assessment forms completed by the two evaluators for all of the studies.

Our worked example revealed a few challenges in assessing transferability. First, the lack of transparency in the reporting of existing economic evaluations, particularly on data inputs (e.g., unit costs/prices), often constrained the ability to determine transferability. The use of the online appendix to provide analytic approaches, and to model assumptions and data inputs in detail, would be valuable. More comprehensive deterministic and probabilistic sensitivity and scenario analyses in published economic evaluations may also help to improve transferability of the external evidence.

Another issue was the inaccessibility of the original models needed to generate results with locally-relevant data inputs. In practice, evaluators

56 Goldman et al.

may reach out to study author(s) to obtain the original model. Access to an original model allows evaluators to revise the analysis, reflecting local data and adapting the model structure or assumptions to be more context-specific. The open-source model would thus be valuable in LMIC settings.[57]

Finally, when assessing interventions and their comparator(s), the feasibility and scalability for Kenya frequently arose as a concern. For example, although many interventions involving diet and exercise counseling are found to be cost-saving or very cost-effective for managing diabetes,[58] it was challenging to assess the availability, feasibility and scalability of such interventions in Kenya without input from a local expert. In actual practice, a diverse set of experts in the evaluation committee, such as epidemiologists, clinicians, disease-program managers and analysts, may help to alleviate some of these concerns.

6.5 Using the Impact Inventory

In previous sections, we sought to provide a framework for decision-makers and practitioners to assess the transferability of economic evaluation to local settings. When possible, analysts should conduct original economic evaluations to identify relevant Best and Wasted Buys in local settings. For these cases, we recommend using an 'Impact Inventory', a structured table listing an intervention's health and non-health consequences, developed by the Second Panel on Cost-Effectiveness in Health and Medicine.[59] The Impact Inventory is intended to ensure that all the consequences of interventions, including those falling outside the formal healthcare sector, are considered regularly and comprehensively (Online Appendix 6D).

Because of the substantial impact of NCDs on non-healthcare sectors, it is essential to consider the potential consequences of interventions for NCDs as much as possible. Ideally, analyses will consider factors, such as health effects on caregivers among Alzheimers patients or the impact of some interventions (e.g., alcohol-use-disorder treatment) on the criminal justice system. Even if decision-makers disagree over how

57 Joshua T. Cohen et al., 'A Call for Open-Source Cost-Effectiveness Analysis', *Annals of Internal Medicine*, 167.6 (2017), 432–33, https://doi.org/10.7326/l17-0695

58 Marseille et al.; Lohse et al.; Bertram et al.; Colagiuri and Walker.

59 Neumann et al.

to value those consequences and do not incorporate them into formal assessments, they should be aware of the potential implications outside the originally intended outcomes in determining an intervention's value. The Impact Inventory provides an approach that allows these components to be considered along with local needs and priorities.

6.6 Conclusion and Next Steps

Identifying locally-relevant Best or Wasted Buys often requires adapting economic evaluations conducted in one country to local settings elsewhere. The process is challenging and requires careful examinations of data inputs, local data availability and other contextual factors relevant to specific settings. The framework and checklist provided in this chapter are intended to be used to assess transferability objectively and transparently in a practical manner. We recognize that others could expand the checklist to include other factors that may be relevant in particular circumstances and we would encourage this tool development. We hope that these tools serve as a useful guide to identifying locally-relevant Best or Wasted Buys.

Improving transparency and reporting in original studies would help an evaluator's ability to assess the transferability of available evidence. Future areas for improving transferability across countries may include multi-national economic evaluations, international cost catalogues (https://ghcosting.org/) and an open-source platform to share decision-analytic models to which local data can be applied. Additionally, future research may examine whether each element of the checklist is equally important for assessing transferability and in what situations it is worthwhile to conduct a thorough transferability assessment considering the resources required for the task.

7. Finding the Best Evidence

Thunyarat Anothaisintawee

7.1 Determining the Impact of Behavior Change on NCDs Through Research

Knowledge changes constantly. For this, if for no other reason, non-communicable disease (NCD) managers must be able to find up-to-date evidence and to interpret and integrate that evidence into their local decision-making. One example is the effect on health of low-calorie sweeteners, as seen in Case Study 7.1.1. Evidence about effectiveness and cost-effectiveness usually come from research findings, so understanding the characteristics, advantages and disadvantages of various types of study design is important for NCD managers if they are to use evidence to good effect in their local contexts.

Case Study 7.1.1 Knowledge growth: A case study of low-calorie sweeteners

Sugar is one of the unhealthiest diet ingredients. Consumption of excessive amounts of sugar can cause diseases like obesity, type 2 diabetes mellitus (T2DM) and heart disease. Despite this knowledge, current intake level is very high. In 2012 the average intake among U.S. adults was 77 grams per day, equal to 19 teaspoons or 306 calories.[1] For this reason, the American Heart Association Nutrition Committee recommended a decrease in added sugar in sweetened products. By

1 Elyse S. Powell et al., 'Added Sugars Intake Across the Distribution of US Children and Adult Consumers: 1977–2012', *Journal of the Academy of Nutrition and Dietetics*, 116.10 (2016), 1543–50.e1, https://doi.org/10.1016/j.jand.2016.06.003

 https://doi.org/10.11647/OBP.0195.07

contrast, low-calorie sweeteners (LCSs) contain few or even no calories while providing an intensely sweet taste. In addition, LCSs do not cause the same metabolic responses in the human body as sugars. These desirable properties make LCSs an attractive substitute for sugar from a public health perspective. LCSs are usually recommended for obese people and T2DM patients in order to reduce their weight and control their blood sugar levels.

However, after using LCSs as substitute for sugar for many years, the shocking evidence from several observational studies was that using LCSs was associated with weight gain and increased the risk of T2DM. These findings were the very opposite of the original belief that LCSs were safe. Despite this evidence, the potential harmful effect of LCSs is debated thanks to inconsistencies in the findings between observational studies and intervention trials. The American Heart Association has recommended against the consumption of LCS beverages by children and encourages the use of water (plain, carbonated and unsweetened) rather than LCSs as an alternative to sugar-sweetened beverages.[2] Based on the available evidence, the potential adverse effects of LCSs are still inconclusive and further research on the association between LCSs and risk of CVDs and cardio-metabolic risk factors is needed.

7.2 Types of Study Design

There are two main types of study design: quantitative and qualitative[3]. A quantitative study is useful for assessing the burden of diseases, exploring the association between potential risk factors and diseases and estimating the benefit of the intervention for the prevention and treatment of diseases. A qualitative study is useful for understanding the process of implementing an intervention, how the intervention works and what the obstacles are to implementing the intervention in practice.

There are several subtypes of quantitative studies[4] as presented in Figure 7.1. Two broad types are experimental and observational. Experimental studies usually allocate subjects randomly into intervention and non-intervention groups (arms of the trial). Such

---

2 Rachel K. Johnson et al., 'Low-Calorie Sweetened Beverages and Cardiometabolic Health: A Science Advisory From the American Heart Association', *Circulation*, 138.9 (2018), e126–40, https://doi.org/10.1161/cir.0000000000000569

3 Leon Gordis, *Epidemiology*, 5th ed. (Philadelphia, US: Elsevier, 2013).

4 Ibid.

studies are called randomized-controlled trials (RCTs). Studies using non-random methods, as when patients are allocated to the arms of a trial according to their birth dates, are called quasi-experimental studies.

Observational studies investigate the relationship between exposures and outcomes. Common types are case-control, cohort and analytic cross-section.[5] If researchers select cases (for example, subjects having interested outcomes) and controls (subjects not having interested outcomes) and compare the odds of exposure between cases and controls, we have a case-control study. If researchers select an interesting group or cohort of the population, measure its exposure or treatment and follow the subjects up until there are outcomes, we have a cohort study. A cohort study usually quantifies the effect of exposure as relative risk, or the probability of the outcome in the exposed group compared with that in the non-exposed group. In analytic cross-sectional studies, researchers select a group of the population, as in a cohort study, but with no follow-up. Exposure and outcome in a cross-sectional study are measured at the same time.

An observational study may be analytical or non-analytical. An analytical study is one that measures a relationship between two variables, like the relationship between interventions or exposures and outcomes. A non-analytical study typically describes characteristics of the population, such as the burden of disease and changes in it, by measuring prevalence and incidence. Descriptive studies commonly consist of case reports, case-series and cross-sectional studies. Analytical studies can be divided into experimental studies, in which researchers assign interventions or exposures to subjects, and observational studies, in which exposure and occurrence of disease are measured as they occur, without experimental controls.

7.3 Quality Assessment of Studies/Evidence

Different study designs have different advantages and disadvantages. RCTs are most free from bias, especially selection bias, because the subjects are assigned to intervention or control groups randomly so that other determinants (confounders) are also randomized.[6] This yields

5 Ibid.

6 Michael Walsh et al., 'Therapy (Randomized Trials)', in *Users' Guides to the Medical Literature: A Manual for Evidence-Based Clinical Practice*, ed. by Gordon Guyatt, Maureen O. Meade and Deborah J. Cook, 3rd ed. (New York: McGraw-Hill Education, 2015).

greater certainty that any difference in outcomes between intervention and control groups is attributable to the intervention rather than other factors. RCT is the most appropriate design for assessing treatment efficacy. However, RCT is not suitable for investigating disease risk factors because it is unethical to allocate subjects randomly to potential harmful exposures. For such investigations, an observational study design is more appropriate. Findings from RCTs cannot always be generalized to non-experimental settings, because the confounding factors controlled for in the trial may be important determinants of the link between causes and consequences in real-world settings. The RCT is highly suited to testing hypotheses about cause and effect, but not so suited to making predictions about outcomes in normal practice. This test is sometimes termed 'internal validity'. Studies that attempt to predict consequences in real-world settings seek 'external validity'.

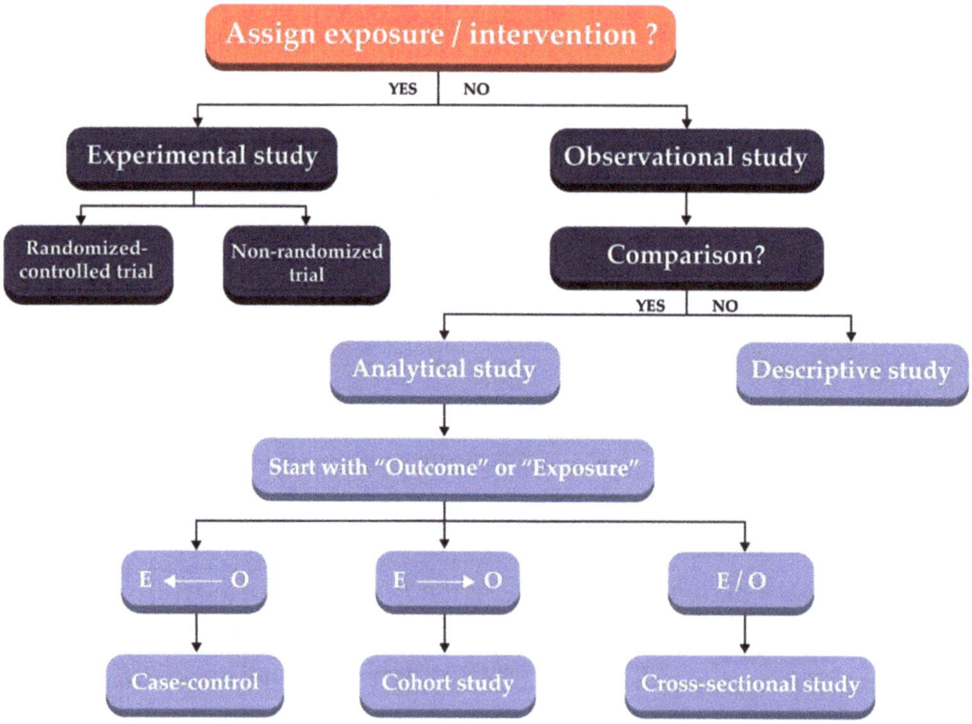

Fig. 7.1 Types of study design.
Note: Outcome = O and Exposure = E.

Observational studies are liable to suffer from confounding bias.[7] This occurs when the measured association between exposure and outcome is distorted by the presence of other factors. These other factors are termed confounding factors or confounders.

Amongst observational studies, the cohort design has the highest validity, because it allows cause to precede effect, so that a temporal relationship between intervention and outcome can be claimed. These studies are, however, time-consuming because of the need to follow subjects up until the outcomes occur. This design is not suitable for rare diseases or for those with a long latent period, such as most cancers.

Case-control and cross-sectional studies can overcome some of the problems with cohort studies because measurements of intervention/ exposure and outcome occur at the same time but the temporal relationship cannot then be understood. Moreover, the case-control design is prone to recall bias because participants are asked to think back to whether or not they received the intervention. People with the disease tend to remember more of the exposure than those without it.

7.4 Types of Evidence Synthesis

Due to the huge and increasing volume of evidence, its synthesis integrates types and sources of evidence into a coherent review. This is called evidence synthesis. These reviews are of two main types, narrative and systematic, as illustrated in Figure 7.2. Systematic reviews have higher validity since its review processes (scope of the review, inclusion/exclusion criteria, selection of studies, data analysis, resolution of disagreements between reviewers) are explicit, transparent and have to be reproducible by other researchers.

Not only have the number of primary researches increased hugely, but the number of systematic reviews has also risen. Many are published every day,[8] so it is impossible for NCD managers or policy-makers to remain up to date with specific topics. Systematic reviews also usually focus on

---

7 Raj S. Bhopal, 'Error, Bias, Confounding and Risk Modification/Interaction in Epidemiology', in *Concepts of Epidemiology: Integrating the Ideas, Theories, Principles and Methods of Epidemiology*, 2nd ed. (Oxford: Oxford University Press, 2008).

8 Hilda Bastian et al., 'Seventy-Five Trials and Eleven Systematic Reviews a Day: How Will We Ever Keep Up?', *PLoS Medicine*, 7.9 (2010), e1000326, https://doi.org/10.1371/journal.pmed.1000326

a specific topic to answer a specific question and so may not provide a comprehensive picture or perspective on complex conditions or problems, which is the usual situation in policy decision-making. For these reasons, umbrella reviews, or overviews of reviews, have been developed. These are tertiary researches that combine data from several systematic reviews that are relevant to a particular health problem.[9] Umbrella reviews apply similar methods to those of systematic reviews but aim to provide a more comprehensive evidence synthesis, by including, for example, evidence of the effectiveness of different interventions for the same condition, or the same intervention for different conditions or populations. The umbrella review is useful for providing a general idea of research in a specific area and also for providing information when the existing evidence about a given topic is inconsistent or contradictory. An example of the umbrella review is presented in Case Study 7.4.1.

A further benefit of umbrella reviews is the speed with which they can be done. For pragmatic reasons, reviews that can synthesize the evidence quickly are likely to be most attractive to NCD managers and policy-makers. Umbrella reviews that consider previous systematic reviews rather than primary researches can save time in work and rapidly provide evidence to inform policy decision-making.

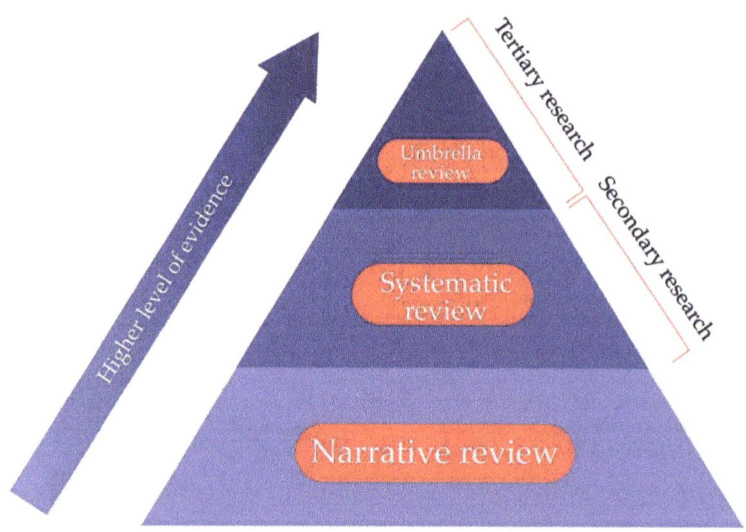

Fig. 7.2 Hierarchy of evidence synthesis.

9 Lisa Hartling et al., 'Systematic Reviews, Overviews of Reviews and Comparative Effectiveness Reviews: A Discussion of Approaches to Knowledge Synthesis', *A Cochrane Review Journal*, 9.2 (2014), 486–94, https://doi.org/10.1002/ebch.1968

Case Study 7.4.1 Efficacy of lifestyle interventions and effect of lifestyle factors on the risk of type 2 diabetes mellitus, cardiovascular diseases and hypertension: An umbrella review

Health-harmful behavior such as eating a poor diet, physical inactivity, inadequate sleep time, use of tobacco and alcohol, all increase the risk of NCDs. Health-harmful behavior also increases the burden of NCDs by increasing their metabolic risk factors, including being overweight/obese, abnormal blood pressure and unhealthy glucose and lipid levels. To prevent and control NCDs, these metabolic risk factors should be reduced by modification of harmful lifestyle behavior. This is an umbrella review of the efficacy of lifestyle interventions for the primary prevention of type 2 diabetes mellitus (T2DM), hypertension and cardiovascular disease (CVD), and the risk effect of harmful behavior (poor diet, physical inactivity, smoking, alcohol drinking and inadequate sleep time) on T2DM, hypertension and CVD. The methods used are in the Online Appendix 7.

Two-hundred and sixty-seven systematic reviews and meta-analyses (SRMAs) of interventions for T2DM, hypertension and CVD met our inclusion criteria and are included in the umbrella review. Of these, 70 were on T2DM, 127 on hypertension and 70 on CVD. Lifestyle interventions considered in the review were diet, physical activity, combined diet control and physical activity interventions, smoking cessation, alcohol drinking and sleep interventions. The effects of each intervention are summarized below.

- Food patterns (e.g., Mediterranean, DASH and diets with high HEI and AHEI scores) reduced the risk of T2DM, CVD and high blood pressure, while the evidence on food groups and food nutrients show conflicting results.
- The findings from this review were similar to those of other reviews and confirm the benefit of moderate and high intensity physical activity in the prevention of T2DM and CVD. However, our review found that low intensity physical activity, such as walking, could also lower the risk of each condition.
- Evidence from systematic reviews and meta-analyses (SRMAs) of RCTs strongly supports the advantage of several lifestyle

interventions in the prevention of T2DM and lowering blood pressure. However, the RCTs showed no significant benefit of lifestyle interventions in the case of CVD.

- There was a J-curve association between alcohol and risk of CVD: moderate but not high alcohol intake significantly decreased the risk of CVD, when compared with non-alcohol intake. However, alcohol reduction in people who regularly drank reduced the risk of T2DM and blood pressure level.
- Sleep is one of the lifestyle factors that was associated with a risk of NCD. People who sleep less than 7 hours/day had significant higher risk of T2DM, CVD and hypertension than people who sleep 7–8 hours/day.

7.5 Role of Environmental Interventions in Changing Health Behavior

The findings from the umbrella review show that health-promoting behavior significantly reduces the risk of developing T2DM. However, encouraging people to change their long-term unhealthy habits and maintain the new behavior for months or years is challenging. Lifestyles are not determined only by individual preferences, but also by sociocultural determinants (i.e., social norms and networks) and environmental influences (e.g., workplace and school environments, city plan and public transport).[10] Motivating people to change their unhealthy lifestyles using only individual-based or health-system strategies might therefore be insufficient to achieve broad success, though applying policy- or population-based approaches by modifying social and environmental factors are likely to be important.

Policy- or population-based interventions target the entire population. These interventions are usually classified into six types:

- behavior-change communication and mass media campaigns,
- front-of-pack labeling and consumer information,
- taxation subsidies and other economic incentives,

10 Johannes Brug, 'Environmental Determinants of Healthy Eating: In Need of Theory and Evidence', *The Proceedings of the Nutrition Society*, 67.3 (2008), 307–16.

- school and workplace interventions,
- local environmental changes and
- direct restrictions and controls.[11]

Policy interventions that are cost-effective by the WHO-recommended cost-effectiveness ratio of ≤100 I$ per DALY averted[12] include: reducing exposure to risk factors such as unhealthy diets and physical inactivity through front-of-pack labelling of salt content, establishment of a supportive environment for lower-sodium options to be provided in public workplace cafeterias and implementing wide public education and awareness of the benefits of physical activity through mass-media campaigns. The status of these measures as Best or Wasted Buys is discussed in Chapters 4 and 5, respectively. Problems in evaluating their cost-effectiveness include the limited nature of the behavior changes actually induced and the time taken for effects to emerge. Additionally, several policy interventions (sugar tax is one) cannot be randomly assigned at the population level, so experimental research designs like RCTs are inappropriate and one needs to turn to natural experimental methods.

Natural experimental studies are called for when an RCT is impractical or unethical, the intervention in question is likely to have a significant health impact but there is uncertainty about its effect size and there is the potential for replication or generalizability of the study.[13] This study design is more susceptible to error through omitted variable bias, loss to follow-up and misclassification of exposure and outcomes. Since the intervention cannot be randomly assigned in the population, this study design affords less protection against selection bias or confounding resulting from selective exposure to the intervention. Explicit multivariate modelling, with accurate measurement of

11 Dariush Mozaffarian et al., 'Population Approaches to Improve Diet, Physical Activity, and Smoking Habits: A Scientific Statement from the American Heart Association', *Circulation*, 126.12 (2012), 1514–63, https://doi.org/10.1161/cir.0b013e318260a20b

12 World Health Organization, *'Best Buys and Other Recommended Interventions for the Prevention and Control of Non-communicable Diseases'*, 2017, https://www.who.int/ncds/management/WHO_Appendix_BestBuys.pdf

13 Peter Craig, 'Using Natural Experiments to Evaluate Population Health Interventions: New Medical Research Council Guidance', *Journal of Epidemiology and Community Health*, 66.12 (2012), 1182–86, https://doi.org/10.1136/jech-2011-200375

exposures, outcomes and potential confounders, in addition to using a large sample size to detect the expected effect, are crucial.

7.6 Conclusion

This chapter has reviewed the armory of research designs that may be called into use in understanding causes and effects in NCD prevention and treatment. The SEED Tool in Chapter 3 recommends systematic reviews or umbrella reviews as useful in answering the fundamental question concerning the theoretical basis of an intervention's effect, which helps to identify both causative variables and potential confounders.

We used an umbrella review of systematic reviews to demonstrate the process of evidence synthesis on the efficacy of lifestyle interventions on health-harming behavior for T2DM, CVD and hypertension. The review process and data synthesis took a long time and required an enormous effort from the review team. Whenever possible, therefore, methods should be modified to accelerate the review process and provide the information to the decision-makers in a timely fashion. In addition, the umbrella review cannot replace policy monitoring and evaluation, since the evidence synthesis is used to inform policy development to identify the most effective intervention. However, monitoring and evaluation of policy implementation remains the key component for ensuring the Best Buy policy.

8. Cross-Sectoral Policies to Address Non-Communicable Diseases

Melitta Jakab and Peter C. Smith

8.1 Introduction

It is well-established that many — if not the majority — of the determinants of health lie outside the immediate control of the health system.[1] The WHO Commission on the Social Determinants of Health[2] collected a vast body of evidence showing that the risk factors associated with poor health arise overwhelmingly from behavioral and social circumstances that cannot be addressed by the health system alone. This insight has led to movements such as 'Health in All Policies', which seek to ensure that health outcomes are given full consideration in all policy areas, including education, housing, transport, environment and fiscal policy. The link between social determinants and non-communicable diseases (NCDs) is especially strong and well-documented.[3]

The importance of other sectors for health-related outcomes has led to a growing interest in the development of cross-sectoral policies to

1 Melita Jakab et al., 'Health Systems Respond to Non-communicable Diseases: Time for Ambition', *Health Systems Respond to Non-communicable Diseases: Time for Ambition.*, 2018, http://www.euro.who.int/__data/assets/pdf_file/0009/380997/Book-NCD-HS.pdf?ua=1

2 World Health Organization, *Closing the Gap in a Generation: Health Equity through Action on the Social Determinants of Health* (Geneva, 2008), https://apps.who.int/iris/bitstream/handle/10665/43943/9789241563703_eng.pdf?sequence=1

3 Michael Marmot and Ruth Bell, 'Social Determinants and Non-Communicable Diseases: Time for Integrated Action', *BMJ (Online)*, 394 (2019), 1251, https://doi.org/10.1136/bmj.l251

 https://doi.org/10.11647/OBP.0195.08

address health objectives. We define the concept of 'sector' broadly, to include both governmental and non-governmental parts of the economy. The only requirement for cross-sectoral working should be that the non-health sector is capable of developing and implementing policies in pursuit of its own sectoral objectives and is prepared to enter into a dialogue with the health sector on matters of mutual interest. Examples include joint working between health and education ministries to improve child health and educational progress, or public-private partnerships to improve the health and productivity of the workforce. It is noteworthy that many reported experiments with cross-sectoral programs seek to target disadvantaged groups and specifically address health inequalities, for which underlying social determinants might be especially important.[4]

The WHO defines *intersectoral action* as 'actions affecting health outcomes undertaken by sectors outside the health sector, possibly, but not necessarily, in collaboration with the health sector'.[5] Using this definition, responsibility for implementing the actions lies outside the health sector, although of course the health sector may be the driving force behind the program and may finance part or all of it. In this chapter we adopt a broader view of collaboration between sectors, which might include but is not limited to the WHO concept of intersectoral actions. Specifically, our definition also includes actions led by the health sector that either have benefits for other sectors beyond health improvement, or where collaboration with another sector is essential for success. An example might be an occupational health intervention that is undertaken by a health system, partly with the aim of improving health *per se*, but also offering potential benefits for employers and the broader economy. We therefore use the term *cross-sectoral* actions in this chapter to describe joint working, whether or not implementation is led by the health sector. This definition of multisectoral actions captures the active collaboration of two or more sectors that deliberately seeks to promote some of the objectives of the health sector.

4 Public Health Agency of Canada and World Health Organization, *Health Equity Through Intersectoral Action: An Analysis of 18 Country Case Studies*, 2008, https://www.who.int/social_determinants/resources/health_equity_isa_2008_en.pdf

5 World Health Organization, *Intersectoral action*, 2019, https://www.who.int/social_determinants/thecommission/countrywork/within/isa/en/

In many cases, cross-sectoral policies are intended to promote the objectives of all the sectors involved and not just those of the health system. For example, an educational policy to promote healthy diets amongst schoolchildren may have an immediate objective for the education sector of improving attendance and performance at school, but may have the additional objective of improving health (and reducing health inequalities) amongst young people. Such effects are sometimes referred to as 'spillovers' of the educational policy. However, the use of this term suggests an incidental (or accidental) benefit for the health sector, with an implication that the education sector would have implemented the program regardless of its effects on health-system objectives. In contrast, in this chapter we are mainly concerned with purposefully designed programs offering joint benefits that might not be implemented without active cross-sectoral collaboration. In such circumstances, the fact that one particular sector may have ultimate responsibility for implementing a program should not disguise its essential cross-sectoral nature.

Many of the NCD interventions discussed elsewhere in this book can be implemented successfully only with the involvement of other (non-health) sectors. It will often be the case that — from a health perspective — such cross-sectoral policies address the risk factors associated with ill-health, rather than specific NCDs. Broad areas of concern include nutrition, sanitation and water quality, air quality, alcohol and drugs, exercise and smoking.[6] The diversity of important risk factors associated with NCDs is an indication of the wide variety of potential cross-sectoral collaborations that might be considered, often addressing the social determinants of health. Note that cross-sectoral work is considered central to the achievement of the United Nations Sustainable Development Goals.[7]

Yet, notwithstanding the manifest importance of cross-sectoral projects for controlling the rise of NCDs, the health sector in many

6 Jeffrey D. Stanaway et al., 'Global, Regional, and National Comparative Risk Assessment of 84 Behavioural, Environmental and Occupational, and Metabolic Risks or Clusters of Risks for 195 Countries and Territories, 1990–2017: A Systematic Analysis for the Global Burden of Disease Study 2017', *The Lancet*, 392.10159 (2018), 1923–1994, https://doi.org/10.1016/S0140-6736(18)32225-6

7 Frank Pega et al., 'The Need to Monitor Actions on the Social Determinants of Health', *Bulletin of the World Health Organization*, 95.11 (2017), 784–87, https://doi.org/10.2471/blt.16.184622

countries has found it difficult to initiate and sustain such working. As we shall discuss, this is in part because of the administrative complexity of managing cross-sectoral projects. But the difficulties are also due in part to limitations in the traditional approach towards evaluating projects that rely on cross-sectoral working. In short, it will usually be the case that cross-sectoral projects need to take account of the objectives of the partner sectors as well as the health sector. We argue that this is not in principle difficult, but does require a reorientation of the cost-effectiveness analysis traditionally applied in the health sector.

The purpose of this chapter is therefore to offer a framework for thinking about the implementation and evaluation of cross-sectoral work to address NCDs. The next section examines the reasons why cross-sectoral work has in many circumstances proved challenging. We then offer a simple analytic framework for assessing the cost-effectiveness of cross-sectoral projects. The fourth section examines the institutional requirements for managing cross-sectoral work and we then briefly present two successful case studies. We conclude by underlining the need for progress in this area if the rise of NCDs is to be successfully moderated.

8.2 Why Are Cross-Sectoral Policies So Challenging?

There is widespread evidence that countries are not exploiting all the opportunities that exist for effective cross-sectoral action to promote health-system objectives.[8] There are many reasons for this. First, it is often extremely difficult to formulate persuasive policies relating to cross-sectoral working. Successful design requires knowledge of all the sectors involved, often requiring novel methods of policy development and knowledge sharing. The various sectors will have different objectives, different budgetary, legal and other constraints and different metrics of success. Reconciling these differences and creating a unified policy is likely to be more challenging than remaining in the 'comfort zone' of single-sector programs.

8 Kumanan Rasanathan et al., 'Governing Multisectoral Action for Health in Low- and Middle-Income Countries', *PLoS Medicine*, 14.4 (2017), e1002285, https://doi.org/10.1371/journal.pmed.1002285; David Mcdaid, 'Institutionalising Inter-Sectoral Action: A Time for Leaping and Pole-Vaulting. *Eurohealth*. 24.1, 13–15.

Second, the institutions of public administration often militate against successful cross-sectoral working. Within government, ministries are usually given discrete budgets, sometimes further constrained by 'budget lines' dedicated to specific services or functions. It is often extremely difficult, or even impossible, to introduce a degree of flexibility into how the budgets are spent. There may in any case be a reluctance to cede some part of a ministry's budget to another sector, as it may be seen to be a signal that the current budget allocation was unnecessarily generous. By spending on cross-sectoral projects, the ministry may fear that in future years its current level of finance will come under threat.

Third, in the same vein, a ministry will usually be judged according to an accountability system that focuses on a narrow set of objectives specific to its own sector. Pursuit of cross-sectoral projects may appear to be diluting its focus on those objectives. Furthermore, if a ministry transfers some of its budget to cross-sectoral activities, it may feel that it loses some degree of control over how the money is spent and the outcomes to be pursued. Existing monitoring systems may be ill-suited to tracking the use of resources and outcomes. Even if good results can be demonstrated, the health ministry may find it difficult to argue that those results are attributable to its own efforts. In short, if cross-sectoral projects appear to sacrifice some degree of control over resources and performance, there may be a reluctance to pursue them. The accountability problem becomes particularly acute when the goals of the partner sector are in direct conflict with those of the health sector — for example, a trade ministry responsible for promoting economic growth may be reluctant to implement taxes on alcohol that could have an adverse impact on (say) the brewing industry.

Finally, implementation of cross-sectoral projects can be especially challenging. Compared with conventional single-sector projects, which have well-established and simple lines of command, a cross-sectoral project may require commitment of resources and authorization from a variety of sources. There may, moreover, be no arbiter to resolve disagreements or accelerate implementation. A potentially effective cross-sectoral project may therefore languish unimplemented, or be poorly implemented, because there is neither the commitment nor the authority amongst the participating sectors to overcome challenges and see the project through to a successful conclusion. In short, the administrative transaction costs associated with cross-sectoral projects may be very high compared to those associated with more conventional projects.

As argued by Rasanathan and colleagues,[9] the fundamental difficulty associated with cross-sectoral projects is one of governance. They argue that 'effective governance is key to the development of shared policy visions and, even more critically, the effective implementation of programs and policies that require coordination across different sectoral agencies and different levels of government'.[10] From the health sector perspective, there has often been a failure to learn from the insights of disciplines such as political economy and public administration, which can offer important lessons for how cross-sectoral working can be pursued successfully. In broad terms, the key requirement for successful cross-sectoral working is what has become known as 'collaborative governance', relying on characteristics such as mutuality, trust and leadership amongst autonomous partners.[11] Such methods are in stark contrast to the conventional 'command and control' models adopted within many ministries.

This chapter is principally concerned with the choice of cross-sectoral interventions to address the prevention of non-communicable diseases. We shall argue that — with minor amendments — cross-sectoral projects can be evaluated using the same cost-effectiveness principles as are customarily used elsewhere. However, it is important to keep in mind the context of governance when considering cross-sectoral projects and to take their feasibility and the costs of implementation fully into account.

8.3 Analytic Framework

The normative principle underlying this book is that cost-effectiveness analysis should form a central pillar for guiding priorities in the prevention of NCDs. As discussed elsewhere, CEA involves estimating the incremental costs to the health system of a proposed intervention

9 Rasanathan et al.

10 Ibid.

11 Kirk Emerson, 'Collaborative Governance of Public Health in Low- and Middle-Income Countries: Lessons from Research in Public Administration', *BMJ Global Health*, 3.Supplement 4 (2018), e000381 https://doi.org/10.1136/bmjgh-2017-000381

and comparing them to the health benefits that would arise, with adjustments for equity considerations if needed. Health benefits will usually be measured in terms of QALYs or their DALY counterparts. Projects should then be ranked according to the chosen cost-effectiveness criterion and any projects with a cost per QALY that is less than the health system's cost-effectiveness threshold should be funded. We assume that the health system's threshold value indicates the maximum the health system is willing to pay for an additional QALY, given its current level of funding.

There has been a great deal of debate in the economics literature concerning the appropriate 'societal' perspective to adopt for evaluating health projects that have consequences (costs or benefits) beyond the health sector.[12] In this chapter we argue that each sector involved in a cross-sectoral project should assess its maximum willingness to pay (WTP) for the project according to its usual evaluation criterion, given the benefits of the project that would accrue to that sector. Then, if the aggregate willingness to pay across the sectors involved exceeds the project costs, the project should go ahead. For the health sector, this means that, when considering contributing to a cross-sectoral project, the same cost-effectiveness principle can be applied to the use of health system funds as is used for conventional single sector projects.

If we know each sector's WTP for the project, based on its specific outcome measures, then we can add these up to obtain the maximum joint WTP for the cross-sectoral project across all the collaborating sectors. If this exceeds the costs of the project, then it should in principle be implemented. The precise funding contribution of each sector to the project will be determined by bargaining and agreement, but the contribution of each sector should be no more than its maximum WTP. In that way, each sector will be participating in a cross-sectoral project that contributes in a cost-effective way to its own objectives. Of course, the bargaining over the precise magnitude of each sector's funding contribution will determine what sort of a Buy (Best, Wasted or Contestable) the project turns out to be for the sector. Fuller details are given in the analytical appendix. This approach is consistent with the 'extended impact inventory' approach

12 Bengt Jönsson, 'Ten Arguments for a Societal Perspective in the Economic Evaluation of Medical Innovations', *European Journal of Health Economics*, 10.4 (2009), 357–59, https://doi.org/10.1007/s10198-009-0173-2

described by Walker et al.,[13] which presents the effects of an intervention across a number of sectoral dimensions, and applies societal values to each dimension to see if the intervention is worthwhile.

Notwithstanding its conceptual simplicity, the usual challenges associated with undertaking persuasive CEA remain when adopting this approach, principally those associated with modelling and quantifying all the relevant health outcome consequences of the initiative.[14] Furthermore, compared with conventional applications of CEA, the benefits of many cross-sectoral NCD initiatives are likely to be distributed across a wide population over a long period, with considerable associated uncertainty. In many cases there is likely to be a need for country-specific epidemiological modelling to identify the impact of NCD initiatives. The need for contextual modelling and the high levels of uncertainty are therefore challenging, However, the principle of using CEA to assess health-sector actions is not altered, even though some of the benefits and costs accrue to other sectors.

The outcomes for one of the partners may be negative for some cross-sectoral projects. This is particularly the case when the health sector seeks collaboration with another sector to create infrastructure that will improve health outcomes. For example, a public-transport initiative might improve access to healthcare facilities and the associated health outcomes. The principle remains the same — the health sector must be prepared to reimburse the transport sector for the necessary opportunity cost this project would impose. However, if the WTP of the health sector exceeds the opportunity cost to the transport sector, then the project should be viable and it should in principle be possible to calculate a financial transfer between the sectors that satisfies both parties.

Some commentators have argued that cost-benefit analysis may be a more appropriate framework than CEA for assessing cross-sectoral projects.[15] Under CBA, the full range of societal benefits and costs arising

13 Simon Walker et al., 'Striving for a Societal Perspective: A Framework for Economic Evaluations When Costs and Effects Fall on Multiple Sectors and Decision Makers', *Applied Health Economics and Health Policy*, 17.5 (2019), 577–90, https://doi.org/10.1007/s40258-019-00481-8

14 Michael F. Drummond et al., *Methods for the Economic Evaluation of Health Care Programmes* (Oxford: Oxford University Press, 2015).

15 Michelle Remme et al., 'Financing Structural Interventions: Going beyond HIV-Only Value for Money Assessments', *AIDS*, 28.3 (2014), 424–34, https://doi.org/10.1097/qad.0000000000000076

from a project would be estimated and monetized. This is a legitimate (though analytically demanding) approach that will demonstrate whether or not — in principle — the project should be implemented from a societal perspective. However, CBA ignores the institutional reality that society has organized much of the economy into discrete sectors (often in the form of government ministries), allocated budget constraints to each sector and attached distinct objectives to the use of those budgets. Furthermore, many cross-sectoral projects entail the involvement of the private (for-profit and not-for-profit) sectors, which may have quite different evaluation criteria from those in the government sector. These institutional constraints in themselves create the need for cross-sectoral delivery of certain projects, because the design of society and government is not aligned with the organizational needs of the project. In these circumstances, CEA is not only a useful device — it is the most appropriate tool for assessing cross-sectoral projects, because it takes into account the financial constraints and missions of each separate sector.

8.4 Institutional Requirements

Once the case for pursuing a cross-sectoral project has been established in principle, an organizational structure for delivering and monitoring the project must be established. As noted above, almost by definition, existing structures of accountability will often be inadequate for this purpose and so some feasible and administratively efficient governance structure must be identified. The design of project governance is mainly beyond the scope of this chapter, but it is important to offer a brief outline of the issues involved in order to give some context to the cross-sectoral case studies that follow.

There are a number of possible models of collaboration for cross-sectoral projects[16]. They include:

- The health sector is the lead actor, but receives support in the form of funding or other resources from an external partner to support the project. The principal governance requirements are proper accountability to the partner for the use of resources and the outcomes achieved.

16 Rasanathan et al.

- The mirror image organizational structure, in which the external partner is the lead actor, but receives support from the health sector. Here the need is for proper accountability to the health sector for the use of resources and the outcomes achieved.
- The health sector is a partner with one or more other sectors to implement projects with joint benefits across the sectors, with a new delivery entity created under the governance of a joint board of control, representing the interests of all partners.
- The health sector is not a formal partner. There is no contribution of resources to the implementing sector, but the health system seeks to influence the implementation and performance of the project in order to promote health system goals (in the spirit of 'health in all policies').

Such modes of working have become quite widespread in some higher income countries and have led to the development of innovative models of management and control, known as 'collaborative governance'.[17] However, such working is less familiar in many LMICs and may require new models of leadership and accountability. For example, a common failing in cross-sectoral projects is a lack of incentives to prioritize the project and a lack of accountability mechanisms to ensure that it is delivered in line with expectations. Although willing to participate, the individual partners may fail to give the project adequate priority because it falls outside their traditional lines of business. Therefore, whatever approach to collaborative governance is adopted, it is likely that the cross-sectoral project will need sustained leadership, often from a very high level of government, to ensure that momentum is sustained and that the outcomes promised by the project are fully realized.

McDaid[18] suggests a number of ways in which incentives can be introduced to strengthen the chosen governance and leadership arrangements. For example:

- the national government (in the form of the finance ministry) can make funds available only if an effective cross-sectoral partnership is put in place;

---

17 Emerson.
18 Mcdaid.

- the national government could introduce a competitive process for funding cross-sectoral projects;
- continued funding of such projects could be conditional on demonstration of successful implementation and evaluation; or
- government ministries could be required to 'ring-fence' part of their budgets for cross-sectoral projects.

Each of these approaches has shortcomings and risks and cannot succeed without appropriate governance and leadership. However, they might serve to underline the importance of cross-sectoral collaboration and emphasize the commitment of the government to such working.

To support the chosen model of governance, there will be a need for information and analysis, in order to monitor implementation and to check that expected outcomes are being secured. This is often challenging because it may be necessary to integrate information systems and reporting requirements from the different sectors. Moreover, it can often be analytically complex to identify the incremental impact of cross-sectoral interventions on expected outcomes. A specific concern in many low-income countries is the large range of often incompatible reporting requirements required by different donor organizations and the preference of such organizations to work in independent 'silos' rather than collaboratively.

Although there have been examples of successful intersectoral projects, few countries have succeeded in institutionalizing cross-sectoral working as a routine undertaking. The UK government experimented with a range of cross-sectoral 'public-service agreements' as a basis for setting ministerial targets and monitoring progress.[19] Under Tony Blair's leadership, a Prime Minister's Delivery Unit was established to drive forward cross-sectoral programs such as childhood obesity reduction.[20] However, this cross-sectoral approach generally failed to take account of its inherent institutional complexity and it lost momentum under subsequent prime ministers. In contrast, the Netherlands has established

19 Peter C. Smith, 'Performance Budgeting in England: Public Service Agreements', in *Performance Budgeting: Linking Funding and Results*, ed. by M Robinson (Washington, DC:, 2007), pp. 211–33, https://doi.org/10.1057/9781137001528_12

20 Audit Commission / Healthcare Commission, 'Tackling Child Obesity — First Steps', 2006, https://publications.parliament.uk/pa/cm200607/cmselect/cmpubacc/157/157.pdf

a Centre for Healthy Living that seeks to promote health by adopting a systematic approach to the evaluation of cross-sectoral policies. An evaluation concluded that the Centre's approach had been 'instrumental in advancing intersectoral health promotion policy and practice across the country'.[21] Finland has an especially successful and long-standing tradition of cross-sectoral health promotion, using instruments such as legislation and administrative reforms at both the national and local level.[22] Even there, however, it has at times proved difficult to nurture a sustained commitment to collecting the evidence necessary to design and evaluate cross-sectoral projects.

8.5 Types of Cross-Sectoral Policies

Whilst it is rare to find cross-sectoral working institutionalized, there are a number of examples of successful cross-sectoral policies in countries at all levels of development. The types of initiatives designed — at least in part — to address NCDs might include, but are not limited to:

- commissioning of non-health infrastructure (e.g., public transport);
- adaptation of non-health programs (e.g., changes to school curriculum);
- sharing delivery platforms (e.g., health sector use of a postal delivery network);
- legislation/regulation affecting non-health sectors (e.g., food labelling);
- taxation or subsidy incentives (e.g., alcohol taxes);
- integrated cross-sectoral programs for specific population groups (e.g., child development programs).

A report of eighteen case studies by the Public Health Agency of Canada and the WHO, albeit focusing on health equity rather than NCDs

21 Nicoline Tamsma et al., *Centre for Healthy Living in The Netherlands: Building Sustainable Capacity and Alliances for Effective Health Promotion* (Copenhagen, 2018), http://www.euro.who.int/__data/assets/pdf_file/0005/365612/gpb-healthy-living-nl-eng.pdf?ua=1

22 Tapani Melkas, 'Health in All Policies as a Priority in Finnish Health Policy: A Case Study on National Health Policy Development', *Scandinavian Journal of Public Health*, 41.Supplement 11 (2013), 3–28, https://doi.org/10.1177/1403494812472296

explicitly, illustrates the wide scope of possible cross-sectoral working and the range of possible institutional arrangements.[23] In this section we present two additional case studies from Hungary and Croatia that entailed legally binding commitments to promote the longevity and effectiveness of the cross-sectoral program.

Case Study 8.5.1. The public catering decree in Hungary: Intersectoral public-health action to improve nutrition and address social inequalities with a binding legal instrument[24]

Context

Addressing obesity, particularly among children, has been a major public-health concern in Hungary to reduce premature NCD mortality and morbidity. Having recognized that voluntary actions alone have not been successful to change unfavorable nutritional outcomes, a complex set of mandatory legal actions have been launched by the Hungarian Government. School catering policies have become the target of action. Because children spend most of their daytime in preschools and schools and 35–65% of their daily energy consumption takes place there, schools have a central role in providing access to healthy nutrition and shaping children's health behavior.

Instrument

A binding legal instrument in the form of a Ministerial Decree was used to increase vegetable/fruit intake and to reduce fat, salt and sugar consumption among school children. The decree came into force on 1 January 2015. Its scope covered pre-schools, primary and secondary schools and other educational settings, inpatient care facilities and certain types of services providing social care and child protection.

The decree gives a definition of nutritious and healthy meals appropriate for age and physiological status and it considers special dietary needs. The decree puts special emphasis on equity by guaranteeing

23 Public Health Agency of Canada and the World Health Organization.

24 http://www.euro.who.int/en/health-topics/Health-systems/health-systems-response-to-ncds/publications/2018/the-public-catering-decree-in-hungary-intersectoral-public-health-action-to-improve-nutrition-and-address-social-inequalities-with-a-binding-legal-instrument-2018

healthy meals free of charge for children in socially disadvantaged families, with the cost covered by public funds. The regulation obliges caterers to provide adequate information to consumers by displaying the amount of nutrients and presence of allergens. A special chapter is dedicated to the mandatory training of caterers.

Making It Happen

The preparatory intersectoral work was led by the Ministry of Human Capacities, a supra ministry covering the areas of health, social affairs, education, youth and sport. Having these various government competencies under one roof facilitated more efficient cooperation, more effective alignment of intersectoral cooperation and a strong social and equity focus included in the decree. The decree was widely and thoroughly negotiated with all relevant stakeholders, including governmental bodies, professional and public organizations (such as caterer associations, parental associations, patient associations and local governments) and with the food industry. Robust communication activities ensured good understanding of public health goals.

Impact

Preliminary evaluations show that between 2013–2017, meals in primary schools became healthier: there was increased consumption of milk and/or dairy products, fruits and vegetables and whole-grain products and cereals and reduced intake of salt and saturated fatty acids. An impact on the food industry was detected in the form of increased willingness to reformulate food with respect to fat and salt content.

Case Study 8.5.2. Employing people with disabilities in Croatia: intersectoral public health action for an inclusive labor market[25]

Context

In Croatia, as in many other countries, people with disabilities are an under-represented group in the workforce. This has a significant impact

25 http://www.euro.who.int/en/health-topics/Health-systems/health-systems-response-to-ncds/publications/2018/employing-people-with-disabilities-in-croatia-intersectoral-public-health-action-for-an-inclusive-labour-market-2018

on their welfare, including their health status, and exacerbates social inequalities in society. People with disabilities account for about 12% of the total population or about half a million people, of which 48% are in the working age group of 19–64 years.

Strengthening employment opportunities for people with disabilities has received growing attention as a civil rights issue and as an under-appreciated growth opportunity for businesses and government budgets. For people with disabilities, employment means greater economic self-sufficiency, an opportunity to use their skills and more active participation in community life. Employment in this group is particularly important because having a disability often means being socially isolated, which negatively influences health outcomes over time.

Instrument

To address this, Croatia implemented a Law on Vocational Rehabilitation and Employment of Disabled Persons in 2013 with the aim of increasing the number of employed people with disabilities.

The 2013 Law focused on regulatory mechanisms including i) quotas related to the number of people with disabilities to be employed, ii) incentives for employers, iii) the development of integrative workshops and working centers which seek to match the abilities of people with disabilities to employment opportunities. The Law also regulates reasonable accommodations to be made at the workplace, including the adaptation of physical barriers and provision of working equipment and personal assistance as needed.

The 2013 law was not an isolated instrument but one component of concerted policy action to support the welfare of people with disabilities, based on prominent regulatory activity developed over 15 years and including more than 250 laws, sub-acts and decisions.

Making It Happen

The role of the Public Health Institute was essential in the development of the 2013 Law and related intersectoral action. It produced evidence-based briefings on the impact of employment policies on the health of people with disabilities and presented them to various working groups that were established to implement the process. The role of producing and presenting actionable evidence proved critical in catalyzing intersectoral action. The Institute also coordinated preparatory action between the various stakeholders to highlight the importance of civil rights and health issues relating to people with disabilities.

Impact

The 2013 Law serves as an effective incentive for employers to hire, recruit and retain people with disabilities. Around 11,000 people with disabilities have been newly employed since the implementation of the Law.

8.6 Conclusions

Many NCD interventions rely on cross-sectoral collaboration for implementation. This chapter has shown that cross-sectoral interventions can — in principle — be analyzed from the perspective of the health sector in the same way that conventional health interventions are assessed, by applying CEA to the health benefits and the costs to the health sector associated with the project. However, cross-sectoral interventions are, by their nature, complex. The evidence to support the analysis will often be in short supply, somewhat speculative or of poor quality. Partner sectors are likely to encounter analogous difficulties when assessing the project from their own perspectives. Therefore, cross-sectoral projects will often need to negotiate serious analytic hurdles before they can even be considered. From the health sector perspective, the role of public health institutes might therefore be crucial in assembling and presenting evidence relevant to the development of cross-sectoral NCD policies.

We have argued that it is difficult to ensure successful implementation of cross-sectoral projects without paying attention to their leadership and governance. To some extent, governance requirements can be met by the suitable design of institutional arrangements, including the specification of the organization responsible for the project, the basis on which it will be held to account and the means of assuring satisfactory performance. Models of collaborative governance are emerging to address such issues, but these are at an early stage of development. There is ample evidence to suggest that any collaborative arrangements must usually be buttressed by a very high level of authority, for example through legislation, or the direct interest of the prime ministerial office.

Notwithstanding these challenges, the importance of the social determinants of health is so great that — without concerted efforts to engage non-health sectors in health promotion — societies will not be able to address the rising burden of NCDs with any effectiveness. Policy-makers therefore need to put in place arrangements for designing appropriate cross-sectoral interventions, assessing their feasibility and performance from the perspective of all the sectors involved, designing appropriate governance arrangements, monitoring the implementation and performance of the initiatives and holding all relevant parties properly to account. This is a major undertaking, especially for the many countries with little experience of such working. However, the potential gains from carefully targeted policies are likely to be very large and the necessary investment in analytic capacity and policy commitment has the potential to transform a health system's approach to health improvement.

8.7 Analytical Appendix

Consider two sectors (say health H and education E) considering a joint project with costs C and joint outputs $b_H > 0$ for health and $b_E > 0$ for education.

First assume that each sector is concerned only with outputs relevant to its own sector. These can be measured in composite measures relevant to the sector, such as (say) additional QALYs for health and additional quality-adjusted years of schooling for education.

Then health would implement the project on its own if and only if $C/b_H \leq k_H$, where k_H is the cost-effectiveness threshold for the health sector;

and education would implement the project on its own if and only if $C/b_E \leq k_E$, where k_E is the cost-effectiveness threshold for the education sector.

In either case, the non-implementing sector would 'free-ride' on the cost-effective project for the other sector.

Suppose now that the project, although producing joint benefits, is not cost-effective for either sector *on its own*. That is, $C/b_H > k_H$ and $C/b_E > k_E$. There might nevertheless still be scope for proceeding if the costs of the project can be shared between the sectors. Given its cost-effectiveness threshold, health should be willing to pay the education sector a side-payment S_H of up to $b_H{*}k_H$ to implement, given the magnitude of the health-related benefits. Education would in turn be prepared to implement if $(C\text{-}S_H)/b_E \leq k_E$; that is if the side-payment is adequate to make the project cost-effective from the education perspective.

Rearranging, this implies $S_H \geq C - b_E{*}k_E$ to assure implementation, with equality to ensure that the project is (just) acceptable to education. A similar argument can be advanced to assess the circumstances under which health would implement the project, subject to a side-payment from education.

Therefore, there is always scope for implementation so long as the project costs C satisfy $C \leq b_E{*}k_E + b_H{*}k_H$, the joint willingness to pay for the project. This requires that health makes a co-funding contribution S_H to education satisfying $b_H{*}k_H \geq S_H \geq C - b_E{*}k_E$. Alternatively, the project could be implemented by health if education makes a co-funding contribution S_E to health satisfying $b_E{*}k_E \geq S_E \geq C - b_H{*}k_H$. This concept can be extended to multiple sectors, or even the general public, when assessing whether a cross-sectoral project can be a Best Buy. Without extending the analysis beyond the health sector, however, we may misinterpret from a societal perspective whether a cross-sectoral project is a Best Buy, a Wasted Buy or a Contestable Buy. Note that in either case the upper limit of the inequality indicates the maximum payment the co-funder would be prepared to make to secure implementation, whilst the lower limit indicates the minimum payment that the recipient would be prepared to receive in order to proceed with the project. The actual choice of S would be a matter for bargaining between the two sectors.

Note that there is no scope for joint implementation if project costs C are such that $C > b_E{*}k_E + b_H{*}k_H$. This means that this cross-sectoral project is a Wasted Buy, even when a broader societal perspective is adopted.

9. Deliberative Processes in Decisions about Best Buys, Wasted Buys and Contestable Buys

Uncertainty and Credibility[1]

Kalipso Chalkidou and Anthony J. Culyer

9.1 Introduction

Deciding whether a prospective buy in the field of Non-Communicable Disease is likely to be a Best Buy is a tricky business. It is tricky for at least the following reasons:

- the criteria for deciding what is a Best or Wasted Buy may not be agreed;
- the alternative best uses of resources (the opportunity costs) are rarely obvious and may lie outside the health sector;
- the health benefits of NCD interventions are often in the long rather than the short term;
- the evidence upon which the appraisal is based is rarely complete, accurate, locally applicable, or entirely relevant and may even be wholly absent;
- the processes through which a decision or a recommendation about a possible Best Buy are made may be secretive,

1 This chapter draws extensively on Anthony J. Culyer and Jonathan Lomas, 'Deliberative Processes and Evidence-Informed Decision Making in Health Care—Do They Work and How Might We Know', *Evidence & Policy: A Journal of Research, Debate and Practice*, 2 (2006), 357–71, https://doi.org/10.1332/174426406778023658; and Anthony J. Culyer, 'Deliberative Processes in Decisions about Health Care Technologies', *OHE Briefing*, No. 48 (2009), https://papers.ssrn.com/sol3/papers.cfm?abstract_id=2640171

 https://doi.org/10.11647/OBP.0195.09

dominated by specific interest groups and incomprehensible to outsiders;

- many of the interventions require collaboration with other sectors and non-health organizations;
- the implementation of any decision is hindered by absent or underfunded delivery mechanisms and organizational weaknesses.

As a result of the foregoing, a decision may lack credibility and generate a mistrust of the professional scientists, clinicians and others involved in the process and bring the use of cost-effectiveness analysis and kindred methods into disrepute.

Each of the recommendations we shall be making can be interpreted as implying the use of deliberative processes in decision making because there will be so much to discuss: the diseases in questions are often insidious in their onset and complex in their manifestation over time; the mix of politics, social value judgments and science is thorough; the disciplines required to understand the interventions and the genesis and treatment of NCDs are in many cases non-medical; the professions involved in diagnosis and treatment are likewise many and include non-medical ones; technical understanding and experience is often limited and needs nurturing with opportunities and support to enable local people to become both competent and confident. There is considerable public interest in finding ways to control the NCD epidemic but less understanding of why the apparent priorities are as they are; in many cases there are vested interests that could be threatened by effective NCD policies but that might be reassured or even brought on side by sympathetic initiatives.

9.2 Criteria, Opportunity Costs and Social Value Judgments: A Role for Deliberation[2]

Everyone involved in NCD prevention and treatment needs to be aware that social values permeate all aspects of both. Decisions are not merely 'technical', let alone scientific. Moreover, since uncertainty abounds,

2 Culyer (2009) offers a series of charachteristics of 'good' deliberative processes; Presidential Commission for the Study of Bioethical Issues, *Deliberation for Better*

all decisions require the exercise of judgment — judgment about the quality of the evidence, the difficulty of implementation, the value of the outcome, the value of what is forgone as resources are committed to specific purposes, the merits of openness and transparency, the worthwhile nature of reaching outside the health and finance ministries, etc. Any criterion for what constitutes a Best Buy embodies value judgments. For example, the commonly encountered 'threshold' criterion, which a technology must meet to be adopted, states that the incremental cost-effectiveness ratio ($\Delta C/\Delta E$) must not exceed a stated monetary sum, thereby making two social value judgments: that cost ought to be a factor and that effectiveness ought to be another. In addition, the threshold criterion embodies an assumption (other things being equal) that more effectiveness is good. Further analysis reveals that effectiveness is typically (though not invariably) indicated by a specific measure such as the Quality-Adjusted Life-Year (QALY) or averted Disability-Adjusted Life-Year (DALY), which may or may not be good proxies for 'health'. Moreover, other things are not always equal, so additional criteria may be required. Two common criteria concern the distribution of health benefits (QALYs or DALYs) and the impact the intervention has on exposure to out-of-pocket costly healthcare needs. Other value-laden issues include how much risk or uncertainty about the evidence can be tolerated; whether future costs and benefits ought to be discounted (reduced in current value) at the same general rate as is used elsewhere in the public sector; how much information (some of which may be claimed to be commercially confidential) should be shared with stakeholders, including journalists and the general public; whether the right technologies have been selected for investigation to start with and for use as comparators; how to negotiate clashes between criteria when they occur; where to look to find out what values the public and its constituents have; and a host of social value judgments regarding the processes of decision-making such as: choice of stakeholders; the nature of their involvement, if any, in decision-making; opportunities to appeal against decisions; the public nature and openness of committee and other meetings and the accessibility of their minutes; the frequency of revisiting past decisions as circumstances and knowledge change.

Health, Science, and Technology Policy: Five Steps for Effective Deliberation 1 (2006) sets out five steps for effective deliberative approaches for decision-making in health science and technology policy.

This list merely elaborates the commonplace observation that 'one size (or recommendation) does not fit all (circumstances)'.

Deliberation is a thoughtful and careful way of reaching a conclusion or deciding something. It is not precipitous and discourages rushed judgments. It involves the focused evaluation of alternatives, weighing their pros and cons. Deliberation can be a learning process — learning about the evidence and learning from other people about perspectives on the question that had not previously occurred to one. In deciding or advising on matters of NCD policy it requires a kind of 'round table' at which significant interests and expertise are represented. A major political value judgment must be made when deciding what counts as 'significant'.

Deliberation can be a means of suppressing the arbitrary and subjective self-interest of the participants in a decision-making process. It should be a means of achieving an impartial state of mind in which people of good will restrain their more selfish personal and professional concerns in pursuit of a wider, or deeper, idea of the social good: one that is not simply the sum of the preferences, prejudices (admirable or not, well-informed or not, representative or not, based on mature reflection or not) of those participating in the debate. Deliberation enables decision-makers to reflect on, discuss openly and possibly revise their beliefs about a problem. Is this our top priority? Who loses most if we do such-and-such? Do we believe the scientists? Can we trust the economists? Have we got the balance between rival assertions right? Have we inferred correctly from the evidence?

9.3 Deliberation Contrasted with Algorithms

In stark contrast to the deliberative process stands the algorithm. An algorithm is a systematic mathematical process sequentially linking various strands in a decision problem to an outcome. A good example of an algorithm for present purposes is the EQ-5D version of the QALY, which combines a set of pre-defined characteristics of good health, measurable at a variety of intensities and weighted in a pre-set fashion in order to measure a health outcome such as the difference between a person's health with and without, or before and after, an intervention or in comparison with an alternative intervention. The algorithm can be made as complicated as one likes, at least in principle, by adding characteristics, breaking it into social subgroupings, refining intensities, changing the weights, including probabilities and uncertainty, discounting future health changes and so on; and every element of the algorithm can even be moderated by the results of consultative engagement with patients, say, for their values, and public health doctors, say, for their beliefs about the transitional probabilities. The process remains, however, mechanical, unidirectional and, if used without interaction between decision-makers, not conducive to learning. Rather than enabling the exercise of judgment about the merits and interpretation of evidence, it can conceal important conclusions that have already been reached. These may (as with EQ-5D) have been reached in earlier (which may even have been deliberative) stages of preparation for a decision, but the nature of dispute resolution, the character of value judgments, the extent of agreement about them, the adequacy of the information base available and so on, all become subsumed in the algorithmic solution. The use of algorithms is likely to be perceived as impenetrable to those not involved in the decision-making process but who may nonetheless have significant stakes in its outcome. The effective use of an algorithm requires there to be sufficient expertise within the decision group for its members as a whole to have confidence that no unacceptable short cuts have been taken. It may often be useful to adopt and then adapt someone else's algorithm. For example, to ensure localization and context sensitivity, several countries have developed their own QALY weighting system.[3]

The same may be said about the use of computerized models to simulate decision-making processes. Computers are good at storing, retrieving, manipulating and communicating information but they cannot exercise judgement. A chair or facilitator and members of the decision-making unit must perform that function: formulating problems, locating those deemed most important, identifying key issues, considering risk and uncertainty about the future, forming preferences, making judgments of subjective value, establishing goals and objectives, appraising the quality of evidence and assessing trade-offs among objectives whilst also incorporating algorithms (and explaining them) into the decision-making process.

3 Richard Norman et al., 'International Comparisons in Valuing EQ-5D Health States: A Review and Analysis', *Value in Health*, 12.8 (2009) 1194–200, https://doi.org/10.1111/j.1524-4733.2009.00581.x; EuroQol Research Foundation, 'EQ-5D-3L | Valuation', 2019, https://euroqol.org/eq-5d-instruments/eq-5d-3l-about/valuation/

9.4 Evidence

Box 9.1 Categories of Evidence

Defined by method of collection, discipline or theoretical framework:

- observational, experimental, quasi-experimental, extrapolated, survey, experiential;
- administrative;
- quantitative, qualitative, economic, ethical/philosophical;
- narrative review, systematic review, meta-analysis;
- legal, epidemiological, clinical;
- clinical epidemiology, decision science, expected utility theory.

Defined by general purpose:

- problem identification, description or scoping;
- cost-containment, efficacy, effectiveness, cost-effectiveness, implementability;
- cultural, leadership, measurement; philosophical-normative, practical-operational; academically driven by discipline (clinical, biostatistics, economics, sociology, etc.).

Defined by source:

- primary research data, secondary data (meta analyses etc.) administrative data;
- clinical experience;
- patient/carer experience;
- political necessity;
- local managerial experience;
- professional (scientific, theoretical, practical, expert, judicial, ethical).

Evidence can be classified in a variety of ways, as summarized in Box 9.1.[4] The first type is based on the *method of collection used* for the evidence; for example, whether it was experimental or from a survey. A second

4 Source adapted from Jonathan Lomas et al., *Conceptualizing and Combining Evidence for Health System Guidance, Canadian Health Services Research Foundation* (CHSRF), (2005).

focuses on the *general purpose* to which the evidence would contribute, such as identifying a problem or measuring the effectiveness of an intervention. A third emphasizes *source*, usually distinguishing research by professional researchers from unsystematic forms of evidence such as 'clinical experience'.

When people in the clinical, management or policy worlds are asked what they consider to be evidence, they tend to think of a medley of scientifically verifiable and locally idiosyncratic types of information, which Lomas et al. call 'colloquial' interpretations, drawing on a wide range of experiences and using a broad definition of evidence.[5] Thus, clinical effectiveness data compete with expert assertion, cost-benefit calculations are balanced against political acceptability and public- or patient-attitude data are combined with the recollection of recent personal encounters with strong personalities. The evidence-informed decision-making movement has, however, engendered for many of them a greater regard for the more scientific forms of evidence than would have been usual thirty years ago and there is an increasing tendency to 'dress up' the conclusions of a decision-making process in the language of science.

By contrast, the research community's view of evidence, both in clinical subjects and the social sciences, tends to be restricted to information generated through a prescribed set of processes and procedures recognized as scientific. In this case, both scientific tradition and more modern influences from the philosophy of science determine what is evidence, which can be summarized as knowledge that is explicit (that is, codified and propositional); systematic (that is, uses transparent and explicit methods) and replicable (that is, it can be tested to see whether others following the same methods with the same samples arrive at the same results).

At a basic level, the general notion of evidence concerns actual or asserted facts (a fact is defined as a 'thing certainly known to have occurred or be true' [Oxford English Dictionary] intended for use in support of a conclusion. Most decision-makers view evidence colloquially and eclectically as anything that increases their degree of belief in a fact (Fig. 9.1). They define it by its resonance with experience and relevance to the

5 Ibid.

kinds of decisions they have to make. This is the first form: colloquial evidence. The second and third forms are two versions provided by scientists. Scientists' views on the role of evidence divide into those who emphasize context-free universal truths (identified closely with evidence-based medicine) and those who emphasize a context-sensitive role for evidence in a particular decision process (identified more with the applied social sciences).

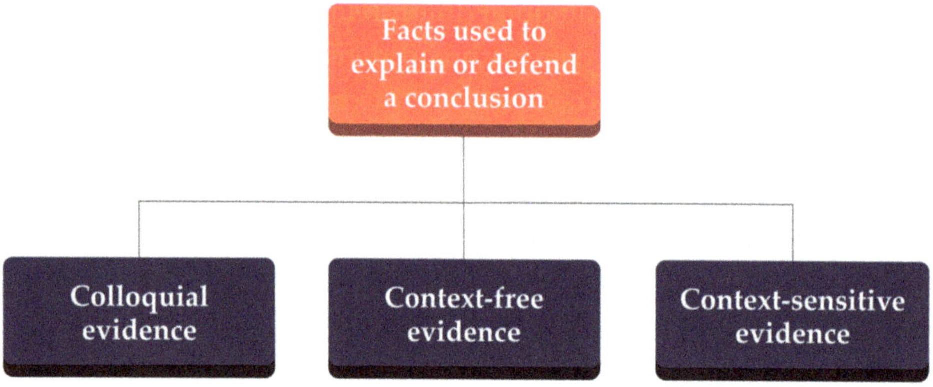

Fig. 9.1 Three different forms of evidence.

The appropriate methods for obtaining scientific evidence about context factors are not the same as those for obtaining evidence related to the testing for the validity of bioscientific hypotheses. Though the research designs may be very different, the scientific principles are, however, the same. Hypothesis testing is common to both, as is the control of 'confounding' variables. But both the phenomena hypothesized about and the method required to do the testing differ. The intent when using context-free evidence is to ensure 'internal validity' of evidence, that is, evidence that is free from bias. The intent when using context-sensitive evidence is to ensure 'external validity' of evidence, that is, evidence that the intervention will work under conditions likely be met in a practical context. Thus, whereas the gold standard procedure for controlling for confounding variables in clinical sciences might be a form of prospective randomized trial, where randomization does much of the work of removing bias from confounders, the gold standard for quantitative social scientists in assessing the resource consequences of adopting a technology is more likely to be a retrospective multivariate econometric study with contextual elements specifically modelled as determinants. Scientific evidence on context must, in addition, be more than merely medical and can embrace professional attitudes, ease of implementation, organizational capacity, competences of workforce, forecasting future burdens of sickness, economics or finance and ethics. Not all will always be relevant, but some will always be relevant (given the context). Colloquial evidence will typically embrace the resources likely to be available, expert and professional opinion on a matter, political judgment, values, habits and traditions, lobbyists and pressure groups and the particular pragmatics and contingencies of a situation. In healthcare decisions, all three kinds of evidence are more or less constantly in play.

These three different forms of evidence — colloquial, context-free scientific and context-sensitive scientific — will not combine of themselves to determine Best or Wasted buys. Combining and interpreting them requires a *process* and the most suitable process may be deliberative through, for example, what has recently been described as qualitative *Multi-criteria Decision Analysis.*[6] Regardless of which of the three types of evidence one is considering, any suitable process needs to address a common set of complexities:

- all evidence needs to be interpreted;
- its relevance needs to be assessed;
- its quality needs to be assessed;
- its applicability in the current context, as compared with that in which it was generated or collected, needs to be assessed;
- its completeness needs to be assessed;
- qualitative evidence needs to be weighed alongside quantitative;
- any technical controversy over its standing needs to be settled;
- the precision of estimates of effectiveness needs to be assessed;
- the robustness of the results needs to be tested by sensitivity analyses;

6 Rob Baltussen et al., 'Multicriteria Decision Analysis to Support HTA Agencies: Benefits, Limitations, and the Way Forward', *Value in Health* 22.11 (2019), 1283–1288, https://doi.org/10.1016/j.jval.2019.06.014

- the evidence, of whatever kind, needs to be considered on the basis of values to determine priorities, 'worthwhileness' and to specify what ought to be done and by whom.

Facts do not 'speak for themselves' and any single piece of evidence, whether of the scientific or colloquial type, is rarely complete enough to enable guidance to be created without further evidence and assessment. To be useful, a deliberative process must therefore facilitate the combination and interpretation of the evidence for the purpose intended and enable those engaged in it to explain why they decided as they did.

Maintaining a common understanding of what constitutes evidence is likely to become increasingly difficult as further interest groups or stakeholders are added in any procedure for determining Best Buys. Conversely, the more homogeneous the group in terms of professional background and level of responsibility, the less tension and disagreement is likely to exist about what constitutes permissible evidence. However, it seems unlikely that the object ought ever to be to maximize the homogeneity merely for the sake of achieving a common understanding. It is convenient if a common understanding can be reached but, if it cannot be reached, then the differences and the reasons for them are worth facing up to explicitly and should not be obscured through selection bias.

In short, the decision-making process ought to provide a means through which the preferences of participants can be transformed rather than merely aggregated; it should be a process that allows participants to change their minds; it should allow the three kinds of evidence to be assessed and combined — colloquial (e.g., from professional experience, case-studies, other gossip); context-free science with high internal validity (such as evidence from explanatory RCTs); context-specific science with high external validity (such as evidence from cost-effectiveness analyses, pragmatic trials,[7] most budget impact analyses) — and it should enable such things that people bring to the deliberation to count (such as their own values, experience, attitudes to risk and degrees of understanding and knowledge).

7 BOLDER research group, 'Better Outcomes through Learning, Data, Engagement, and Research (BOLDER) ? A System for Improving Evidence and Clinical Practice in Low and Middle Income Countries', *F1000Research*, 5 (2016) 693, https://doi.org/10.12688/f1000research.8392.1

Some of the problems posed by evidence that might be resolvable through deliberation include situations where:

- evidence from more than one expert discipline is involved;
- evidence from more than one profession is involved;
- some stakeholders' interests are threatened by evidence;
- there are technical disputes to resolve;
- evidence is scientifically controversial;
- evidence is incomplete;
- evidence is lacking;
- evidence gathered in one context is to be applied in another;
- issues of outcome, benefits and costs go beyond the conventional boundaries (of concept and end-point) of medical research design;
- there is substantial uncertainty about key values;
- there are risks (quantified or unquantified) to patients that need to be assessed and weighed;
- there are risks (e.g., of malpractice suits) to professionals that need to be assessed and weighed;
- there are other social and personal values not taken into account in the scientific evidence;
- there are issues of equity and fairness of treatment (e.g., of patients similar in many respects but differing in their capacity to benefit);
- there are issues of implementability and operational feasibility;
- there are issues of short-term financial feasibility;
- there are reasons to suppose that implementation may seriously destabilize local strategies and priorities;
- wide professional 'ownership' is desired;
- public credibility is desired;
- political 'trust' is involved (e.g., no unpleasant surprises for ministers; help on how to handle unwelcome or embarrassing evidence).

When there is evidence from more than one expert discipline, issues can easily arise about language. 'Cost' and 'outcome' are unlikely to mean the same to a clinician, a sociologist or an economist. Confusion may arise through failing to distinguish between statistical, clinical and policy significance. Views about the relative virtues of cross-sectional and time-series data are not shared. Bayesians and frequentists do not always see eye to eye. Equilibrium gets confused with equipoise. There are a lot of conventions that are manifestly different between disciplines and these can easily become barriers to communication. Many such issues can be resolved only by talking and, moreover, by frequent engagements of a deliberative character.

Feeling threatened is something that is dangerous, not only for the person threatened but also for the whole decision-making process. A deliberative process can be one in which people's interests are exposed and the character of the risks to which they are exposed is assessed. That in itself may be sufficient protection, for example, through enabling those affected to take preliminary steps to minimize adverse impacts, or for further analysis of the size of the threat and for exploration of any more extensive protection or compensation that might be warranted. But further protection may be required if, say, the revelation that a member of a committee espoused an unpopular political position were to lead them to subsequent discrimination and harm.

Deliberation is likely to be useful when there are technical disputes to resolve in connection with evidence. These are endemic and non-trivial. Some relate to the evidence itself, some to its generation and some to the methodology used to summarize it.

Complex problems will often benefit from deliberation. Examples include issues concerning outcomes, benefits or costs, any or all of which might go well beyond someone's conventional boundaries of concept (for example, when the principal beneficiary is a family member rather than the patient); issues of metric (biological proxy measures of outcome like blood pressure in comparison to the clinical or social consequences of such indicators); issues of end point (end of trial versus remainder of expected life); issues of uncertainty about the importance attached to different elements in a decision; and lots of other types of issue too.

9.5 Uncertainty

Uncertainty is all-pervading, both that which is formally measured through conventions about statistical significance (for example, less precision in an estimate is usually indicated by a larger standard error) and that which is qualitatively expressed, for example, via a Likert scale of 'more or less' likelihood. There can be uncertainty about the right methodology (should benefits be discounted by the same factor as costs? Was the sample large enough to make statements with confidence about the experience of subgroups of patients? Was the measurement of other social and personal values, which are not normally taken into clinical account, appropriate? Ought such effects be taken into account at all?) It seems plausible to suppose that open discussion about matters of which one is uncertain may help to locate more precisely the reason for the uncertainty and whether, for example, it is the sort of uncertainty that can be resolved by having more, or better, data; or that needs greater investigation of analytical methods; and whether there is a comfort in agreeing on a course of action about which there is a consensus, even though everyone is uncertain. When taking politically controversial decisions, it may be helpful for the minister to be able to explain in Parliament and to the public that there has been extensive consultation, much deliberation, full consideration of expert opinion and the ample weighing of the values of those most affected by the decision. At a minimum, the case becomes easier to make that the decision was not arbitrary and its rationale becomes communicable. This will take on specific significance if the decision is an unpopular one. *Both* the process *and* its outcome help to make a decision credible and to legitimize it.

9.6 Credibility

Decisions taken on behalf of other people need to be credible. That is, the 'other people' in NCDs, typically the public at risk and the professionals who care for them, want to know that decisions taken were taken for good and understandable reasons (especially when controversial); that they were taken in a way consistent with generally accepted social values; and that they were informed by the best quality evidence available. This is true not only of decisions regarding Best Buys but also, and perhaps especially, of buys judged likely to be Wasted, especially if such buys have powerful political or commercial backing. If the public is going to be able to judge the credibility of the decisions made on its behalf, it needs to be able to penetrate the decision-making process to discover whether the reasoning was sound (and other possible decisions considered); the value judgments were acceptable; and whether the evidence was appropriately identified and interpreted. The public will want to be satisfied that those involved in the process were competent (for example, that the scientists were men and women of unimpeachable scientific authority and integrity); that they sought to promote the public interest and not a narrow selfish interest (whether personal, professional or commercial); and that those who were there to represent the public were appointed in a fair way and could be held to account. Credibility is further served if all stakeholders (i.e., any group likely to be affected for good or ill by the decision) have had a reasonable opportunity to comment before a final decision is taken.

Deliberative processes often include, but are not the same as, consultation or comment. A famous example of consultation was the Oregon experiment to help determine which clinical procedures ought to be included in that state's Medicare program. It was not a deliberative process, but a process of consultation in which there were forty-seven community meetings, twelve public hearings and fifty-four panel meetings for healthcare providers. All the data thereby gathered was fed into a committee (the Oregon Health Services Commission) for prioritization of procedures.[8] Thus, many were *consulted* prior to the decision but relatively few *participated* in its making. The Commission itself doubtless engaged in much deliberation but the participation of all those people who were consulted was not part of the decision-making.

Nor are opportunities to comment the same as deliberation. The National Institute for Health and Care Excellence in England and Wales (NICE) provides opportunities for people to comment on technologies that are under appraisal, alongside consultation and deliberation. The public in general might be invited to comment (say, via a website) and

8 Michael Garland, 'Rationing in Public: Oregon's Priority-Setting Methodology', in *Rationing America's Medical Care: The Oregon Plan and Beyond. Brookings Institution*, ed. by M. A. Strosberg et al. (Washington, DC: Brookings Institution, 1992).

some individuals or organizations may receive specific invitations. Like consultation, commenting can be a part of a deliberative process, but it is not to be equated with one. Neither consulting nor commenting involves mutual deliberation. There is limited interchange, there is restricted participation and neither is an arrangement for the actual taking of decisions, whereas deliberative processes can embody all three. This is what makes deliberative processes different.

One approach that embraces the whole range of comment, consultation and deliberative participation is the Cooperative Discourse Model.[9] This entails the elicitation of values and criteria from stakeholder groups, the provision of policy options by expert groups and the evaluation and design of policies by randomly selected citizens. This was a model that seems to have been used to good effect by the UK Committee on Radioactive Waste Management, which is an independent committee established by the UK Government in November 2003 to develop recommendations for the long-term management of higher level radioactive wastes and which faced a classic set of issues of science and of value. Its terms of reference explicitly required that the review

> be carried out in an open, transparent and inclusive manner [...] must engage members of the UK public, and provide them with the opportunity to express their views. Other key stakeholder groups with interests in radioactive waste management [...] [had also] to be provided with opportunity to participate. The objective of the review [was] to arrive at recommendations which can inspire public confidence and [were] practicable in securing the long-term safety of the UK's radioactive wastes. It must therefore listen to what people say during the course of its work and address the concerns that they raise.[10]

The use of the Cooperative Discourse Model seems to have been a success — at least as judged by the criterion that the client knows best. The Government's response to the report included this:

> The reflection of a wide range of viewpoints, and a basis in sound science is key to providing recommendations which inspire public confidence for managing the wastes in the long term, providing protection for

---

9 Ortwin Renn, 'A Model for an Analytic–Deliberative Process in Risk Management', *Environmental Science & Technology*, 33.18 (1999), 3049–55.

10 Committee on Radioactive Waste Management, *Managing Our Radioactive Waste Safely* (London, 2006).

> people and the environment. The open and transparent manner in which CoRWM has conducted its business has been ground breaking. Accordingly, Government welcomes CoRWM's report and believes it provides a sound basis for moving forward. Most recommendations can be acted on immediately; others require us to undertake more work.[11]

The production of evidence itself will often have embodied deliberative processes as, for example, in scientific discussions of the design of a research project, clinical trial or systematic review. The typical scientific evidence on (context-free) efficacy is summarized in the form of narrative reviews, systematic reviews or meta-analyses (each of which will themselves have involved a lot of 'judgment') and each of which in itself will have often embodied mini-deliberative processes. Thus, within deliberative processes lie further deliberative processes. 'Artificial' evidence, such as evidence from economic/epidemiological models that extrapolate beyond experimental time periods, is particularly suited to deliberation, as is the evidence that comes up through colloquial processes like public meetings, hearings from special witnesses and survey material.

No evidence is totally authoritative; it all involves judgments by people in its creation, assembly and presentation. Some of the judgments are technical and scientific (was the most efficient estimating procedure used?). Some are scientific but also interpretive (are the trial results applicable in another setting?). Some are scientific and judgmental (were the scientists at risk of bias from their funding sources?). Some have the character of social value judgments (was the outcome measure an appropriate indicator of health?). Moreover, these are all questions about which it is perfectly possible for both scientifically trained and lay people to disagree amongst themselves. To be credible, therefore, all these judgments need to be seen to have been reasonable under the prevailing circumstances.

---

11 UK Government, *Response to the Report and Recommendations from the Committee on Radioactive Waste Management* (CoRWM) *by the UK Government and the Devolved Administrations* (London, 2006).

9.7 Some Characteristics of Deliberative Processes

The table below[12] offers some specific practical examples of how some common features of deliberative processes can be given a practical form.

Table 9.1 Principles of good governance for HTA.

Principles	**Examples of how bodies can adhere to these principles**
Independence	Maintain arm's length from government, payers, industry and professional groups; Strong and enforced conflict of interest policies.
Transparency	Meetings are open to the public; Material placed online; decision criteria and rationale for individual decisions made public.
Consultation	Wide and genuine consultation with stakeholders; Willingness to change decision in light of new evidence.
Scientific basis	Strong, scientific methods and reliance on critically appraised evidence and information.
Timeliness	Decisions produced and published in a reasonable timeframe.
Consistency	The same technical and process rules are applied to all priority-setting channels.
Regular review	Regular updating of decisions and of methods, with review dates specified in final reports.
Contestability	The decision-making process can be challenged, through legal challenges or non-judicial appeal mechanisms.

We are not advocating the indiscriminate use of deliberative processes. They are costly and may not be worth their cost. In LMICs, in particular, gaining credibility may present challenges that are hard to overcome, such as the availability of sufficiently qualified and independent individuals or the availability of evidence of direct local relevance. Under such

12 Reproduced from Francis Ruiz, Kalipso Chalkidou and Laura Morris, 'Process Matters for Priority Setting and Health Technology Assessment in Indonesia', *F1000Research*, 8 (2019), https://doi.org/10.7490/f1000research.1116839.1

circumstances, the transparency of the decision-making process becomes even more important, if the client population is to believe that what is claimed as a Best Buy is truly likely to be one and that interventions deemed to be Wasted Buys really are inferior to the alternatives.

In the early days of the life of an advisory or decision-making organization that is to determine Best Buys, in-camera sessions might be used more frequently than in its more mature days, because at least some members might feel intimidated by the presence of a public, or afraid of unpleasantness downstream should their support for a decision lead to an unwanted outcome, or simply wish to avoid looking indecisive because they have changed their mind about something. Other participants (local politicians, aggressive lobbyists, show-off clinicians) may play to the crowd. Plainly, such measures will militate against credibility, so conflict between the ideal and the practical should be minimized as much as possible. For example, minutes could record disagreements without naming names, meetings could be held with only a select group of public witnesses present and absent evidence could be replaced with the best possible local or international expert opinion.

9.7.1 Case Study: The (then) National Institute for Clinical Excellence (England and Wales)

NICE was created to be an authoritative foundation of 'clinical governance'. This was (and is) a framework through which National Health Service (NHS) organizations are accountable for continually improving the quality of their services and safeguarding high standards of care by creating a local environment for managing accountability and the audit of clinical practice. From the beginning, it was decided that NICE's procedures would be conducted with the highest degree of transparency possible and with much participation by 'stakeholders'. These were categorically defined as patients, informal caregivers, clinical and other professional caregivers, healthcare managers, manufacturers, researchers and the public in general. NICE insisted on being located within the NHS rather than the Department of Health (ministry). It sought the respect of the overwhelming majority of the country's clinical-and-health-service research community and the support of the Royal Colleges of Medicine and other bastions of professional life. The royal colleges are the principal professional associations of the United Kingdom's medical professions. They comprise: The Royal College of Anesthetists, The Royal College of General Practitioners, The Royal College of Obstetricians and Gynecologists, The Royal College of Pediatrics and Child Health, The Royal College of Pathologists, The Royal College of Psychiatrists, The Royal College of Radiologists, The Royal College of Surgeons of England, The Faculty of Public Health Medicine, The Faculty of Pharmaceutical Medicine and The Faculty of Occupational Medicine.

It was important to NICE that its guidance could not be dismissed as cranky, under-researched, or second rate. But it also had to be acceptable to the NHS's users and fair to the inventors and manufacturers of the various interventions in a huge range of patient-management pathways. It also had to be deemed 'do-able' by the managers. There had to be lots of opportunities for skeptics and any who might feel threatened to air their concerns and for NICE to respond appropriately.

Some of the ways in which NICE sought to be a model of deliberative process were:

- there were open Board meetings that took place bi-monthly around England and Wales, accompanied by public receptions and 'Question and Answer' sessions with the chair;
- minutes were published on the NICE web pages before confirmation by the Board;
- there was a Partners' Council. This had a statutory duty to meet once a year to review NICE's annual report. In practice, in the early days it met more frequently as a source of advice and a forum for exchanging ideas and developing the future plans for the Institute. Its membership included representatives from organizations with a special interest in its work such as patient groups, health professionals, NHS management, quality organizations, industry and trade unions. Members were appointed by the Secretary of State for Health (English minister) and the Welsh Assembly Government. It was abolished after a few years having served a useful function in getting NICE respectably off the ground;

- there was a Citizens' Council. This was a form of 'citizens' jury' that considered social-value-laden matters referred to it by the Institute's Board. Its thirty members had no economic involvement in the healthcare system and were selected to representative of the regions and demographic characteristics of England and Wales. Members were paid £150 per day plus their travel and subsistence expenses. It met twice a year and adopted a deliberative approach and could call witnesses and commissions papers. It was managed at arm's length from NICE by a company specializing in research and community consultation;
- the membership of the Technology Appraisals Committee was set broadly. The Committee was a standing advisory committee of the Institute, which had a very public profile since it was the source of NICE's recommendations for the NHS. Members were appointed for a three-year term. They were drawn from the NHS, patient and care-giving organizations, relevant academic disciplines and the pharmaceutical and medical devices industries. Names of Appraisal Committee members were posted on the Institute's website;
- there were extensive consultation exercises throughout the appraisals process;
- there was an appeals procedure. There were three grounds for appeal: that the Institute had failed to act fairly and in accordance with the Appraisal Procedure set out in its Guidance to Manufacturers and Sponsors; that it had prepared Guidance which was perverse in the light of the evidence submitted; and that it had exceeded its legal powers;
- there were consultative processes about process. For example, the process through which the procedures for health technology assessment were developed involved several committees with representation of experts from a variety of stakeholders. The outcome was a public document describing procedure;[13]

---

13 National Institute for Clinical Excellence, *Guide to the Methods of Technology Appraisal* (London, 2004).

- there were extensive liaisons with eleven Royal Colleges, seven Independent Academic Centres and seven National Collaborating Centres. NICE created the National Collaborating Centres within consortia that consisted of the royal colleges, professional bodies and patient/carer organizations for developing clinical guidelines. They were: the National Collaborating Centres for Acute Care, Cancer, Chronic Conditions, Mental Health, Nursing and Supportive Care, Primary Care and Women and Children's Health;
- there was considerable joint working with NHS R&D and the National Coordinating Centre for Health Technology Assessment. This was a part of the Wessex Institute for Health Research and Development at the University of Southampton. It coordinated the national HTA research program on behalf of NHS R&D.

Thus, it was determined that the process of technology appraisal was to be open, multi-disciplinary, multi-professional and multi-institutional and that it would have 'lay' participation. It was heavily dependent upon people's willingness to serve pro bono. It was plain from the outset that very large numbers of people would be involved and the Institute itself would be largely a virtual organization.[14]

Several of these features have been modified since 1999, mainly on grounds of expense, and it is easy to see that NICE, as a 'Rolls Royce' of such institutes, cannot be a model to be adopted wholesale anywhere else, nor has it survived as such in England and Wales. Its features, however, facilitated deliberation in evidence-informed decision-making and can readily be adapted to suit different contexts.

9.8 Conclusions

A deliberative process for selecting Best Buys is likely to:

- identify relevant clinical, social and political contexts for interpreting context-free scientific evidence about NCDs,

14 Anthony J. Culyer, 'NICE's Use of Cost Effectiveness as an Exemplar of a Deliberative Process', *Health Economics, Policy, and Law*, 1.Pt 3 (2006), 299–318, https://doi.org/10.1017/s1744133106004026

simply by virtue of the fact that representative people and people who can interpret the scientific evidence on external validity are there at the table;

- generate guidance that is consistent with the context-free scientific evidence and its reasonable interpretation in particular contexts;
- command a wide credibility in professional circles and beyond, simply because respected professionals are there at the table;
- result in a quality and power of residual opposition that is low. The prediction is that there will be less hurt, less offence and therefore less opposition if deliberation is used than without it;
- result in less alienation. If the process is one whose design was actually shaped by everybody with a stake in its outcome, so that they actually become parties to its design and committed to the nature of the process, stakeholders are much less likely to be alienated by its outcome. After all, it was a process that they helped to design and even approved, rather than some other arbitrary process that somebody else invented and thrust upon them. They are more likely to be able to live with the consequences of deliberation, even if on occasion the approved process produces results that are not their preferred ones;
- generate guidance whose implementation will be speedy;
- identify impediments to the implementation of guidance and to find solutions to those impediments: ways of leaping over or going around them;
- identify knowledge gaps that might be resolved by further enquiry and research.

Finally, deliberation is not about establishing consensus. There is a lot to be said, however, for discovering whether there is or is not consensus and, when there is disagreement, whether it is a matter of fact that might be resolved by further research and other factual enquiry, a matter of methodology or procedures which might be resolved by specialist workshops, or a matter of value which may need a political resolution at a high level. The important principle to keep in mind is that of facing up to difficulties rather than burying them and of demonstrating reasonableness in the ways they are handled. Therein lies credibility.

10. Summing Up

Wanrudee Isaranuwatchai, Rachel A. Archer and Anthony J. Culyer

The global community has to reckon with the scourge of non-communicable diseases (NCDs).

In an ideal world, it would be easy and straightforward to prioritize and allocate resources to interventions that have the maximum impact on health, while ensuring fair distribution of resources to all and minimizing the risk of financial hardship from out-of-pocket payments. In the real world, however, things may be quite different. Some may be opposed to allocating healthcare resources according to impact and fairness (they have their own agendas); there is evidence but it is patchy and not always agreed by the experts; sometimes that evidence may not be suited to 'our' situation; sometime there is simply no evidence at all. There are other uncertainties: do we have the resources to make a real impact; are our methods good enough; can we train up enough people with the right skills; can we institutionalise the necessary expertise; and can we find ways of making complicated matters accessible to public understanding? In the real world, things may not be perfect, they may not be ideal but it is our world. It is the world that is continuously challenged by the burden of NCDs.

In this book, we have tried to bring the two worlds together. We have made a number of suggestions for mitigating some of these difficulties and enhancing the ability of societies to address the rising burden of NCDs more effectively and efficiently. We have provided definitions of commonly used terms and some basic theory drawn from the literature on effectiveness and cost-effectiveness encompassing the fields of

 https://doi.org/10.11647/OBP.0195.10

epidemiology and economics. Specifically, we have presented some ideas and tools to help decision-makers and NCD program managers in 'NCD Units' to navigate this complex landscape. These ideas include but are not limited to:

- creating organizational structures that facilitate multisectoral approaches (Chapter 2);
- creating authoritative guidance at the global level to impact effectively on political leadership and at the local level for NCD program managers (Chapter 2);
- introducing Systematic thinking for Evidence-based and Efficient Decision-making (SEED) as a tool for evaluating the evidence base — a thinking aid with step-by-step practical considerations to implementing Best Buys and avoiding Wasted Buys (Chapter 3);
- using a list of Additional Considerations to supplement cost-effectiveness analysis and to complement SEED (Chapter 4);
- sharing real-world case studies of Best Buys, Wasted Buys and Contestable Buys (Chapters 4 and 5);
- working systematically and in a participatory manner with stakeholders (Chapter 5);
- providing a means of effective interrogation of claims that particular buys are Best Buys through descriptions of some common characteristics of inefficient spending (Chapter 5);
- using realistic thresholds and selective implementation strategies (Chapters 5 and 9);
- using the Transferability Framework and Checklist for assessing the applicability of research results obtained elsewhere (Chapter 6);
- cultivating awareness of the strengths and weaknesses of different research designs with real-world examples on the efficacy of lifestyle interventions on health harming behavior for type 2 diabetes, cardiovascular diseases and hypertension (Chapter 7);

- devising accountability and governance arrangements that match multisectoral requirements (Chapters 8 and 9); and
- understanding that one size seldom fits all in a health care system, especially across countries (throughout).

Key learnings and practical frameworks (the SEED Tool, transferability checklist, etc.) also have potential beyond NCDs and, indeed, across the whole fields of public and personal healthcare and of non-healthcare that impacts on health (the environment, education, housing and so on). These are topics for future research. While this book cannot solve all problems related to the political economy of NCDs, it does offer key considerations and guidance for assessing and implementing NCD interventions. We are not denying that there is a long road ahead and that universal problems may lack universal solutions. We know full well that prevention is often seen as the poor cousin of treatment and that budgets often have no room for it. Program managers usually find themselves navigating systems with inappropriate disease-focused structures and decisions frequently need to be made in the absence of good quality local evidence. However, there are also lessons we can learn from other countries and there are methods we can employ to assess the applicability of other countries' evidence.

Buys, in the case of NCD prevention, are often complex, constantly changing and unique to each jurisdiction. There is no 'one-stop shop' for policy-makers, but there are positive steps we can take to continue our efforts to support NCD prevention. This work has been a guide to some of the more important ones.

Glossary of Abbreviations

AHEI	Alternate Healthy Eating Index
BMJ	British Medical Journal
BTT	Benefit-based tailored treatment
CE	Cost-effectiveness
CEA	Cost-Effectiveness Analysis
CD	Communicable diseases
CHEERS	Consolidated Health Economic Evaluation Standards
CONSORT	Consolidated Standards Of Reporting Trials
CVD	Cardiovascular diseases
DALY	Disability-adjusted life-year
DASH	Dietary Approaches to Stop Hypertension
DCP	Disease Control Priorities
DIY	Do It Yourself
EQ-5D	EuroQol 5-dimensional questionnaire
EQUATOR	Enhancing the QUAlity and Transparency of Healthcare Research
EURONHEED	European Network of Health Economics Evaluation Databases
FCTC	Framework Convention on Tobacco Control
GEAR	Guide to Health Economic Analysis and Research
GDP	Gross Domestic Product
GH	Global Health

HIAS	Hitotsubashi Institute for Advanced Study
HITAP	Health Intervention and Technology Assessment Program
HEI	Healthy Eating Index
HLC	High-level Commission
HTA	Health Technology Assessment
I$	International dollars
ICER	Incremental cost-effectiveness ratio
iDSI	international Decision Support Initiative
IOM	Institute of Medicine
ISPOR	International Society for Pharmacoeconomics and Outcomes Research
JICA	Japan International Cooperation Agency
KEMRI	Kenya Medical Research Institute
LCSs	low calorie sweeteners
LMICs	Low- and middle-income countries
NCD	Non-communicable diseases
NPP	NCD Prevention Project
NICE	National Institute for Health and Care Excellence in England and Wales
NHS	National Health Service (United Kingdom)
OECD	Organization for Economic Co-operation and Development
PAHO	Pan American Health Organization
PEN	Package of essential non-communicable disease interventions
PMAC	Prince Mahidol Award Conference
PMAF	Prince Mahidol Award Foundation
PRICELESS SA	Priority Cost-Effective Lessons for System Strengthening in South Africa
PRISMA	Preferred Reporting Items for Systematic Reviews and Meta-Analyses
QALY	Quality-adjusted life-year

RCT Randomized controlled trial

RCSC Royal Civil Service Commission

SEED Systematic thinking for Evidence-based and Efficient Decision-Making

SF-6D Short-Form Six-Dimension

SSB Sugar-sweetened beverage

STROBE Strengthening the Reporting of Observational Studies in Epidemiology

THF Thai Health Promotion Foundation

T2DM Type 2 diabetes mellitus

TTT Treat-to-target

UK United Kingdom

UN United Nations

US United States

USAID United States Agency for International Development

USD US dollars

WHO World Health Organization

WTP Willingness-to-pay

List of Illustrations and Tables

Chapter 1

Chapter 2

Chapter 3

Chapter 4

Chapter 5

Chapter 6

Chapter 7

Chapter 9

End page

www.ingramcontent.com/pod-product-compliance
Lightning Source LLC
LaVergne TN
LVHW082230200926
848484LV00008B/2329